Aiming at Medicine?
Human Biology, Health Science and Medicine Futures

How a Student became a Doctor?
Why a Physician left Practice for Research?
What a Professor did?
What a Dean couldn't?
Will you, New Students, help strengthen your Futures?

I want these questions to be useful:
To students, dreaming of human biology, health science,
and medical futures,
To parents (especially doctors and scientists) wondering
if students should follow them,
To grandparents, proud of grandchildren,
whatever they want to do,
To anyone, interested in the combination of teaching,
discovery, practice and service,
And to everyone, fearing today's regress,
wanting tomorrow's progress

Charles Oxnard

Acredita No Veio: Listen to the Old Man
(The words of Edson Arantes do Nascimento, Pelé)

AIMING AT MEDICINE?

Human Biology, Health Sciences
and Medicine Futures

Charles Oxnard

University of Western Australia, Australia

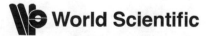

NEW JERSEY · LONDON · SINGAPORE · BEIJING · SHANGHAI · HONG KONG · TAIPEI · CHENNAI · TOKYO

Published by

World Scientific Publishing Co. Pte. Ltd.

5 Toh Tuck Link, Singapore 596224

USA office: 27 Warren Street, Suite 401-402, Hackensack, NJ 07601

UK office: 57 Shelton Street, Covent Garden, London WC2H 9HE

British Library Cataloguing-in-Publication Data
A catalogue record for this book is available from the British Library.

AIMING AT MEDICINE?
Human Biology, Health Sciences and Medicine Futures

ISBN 978-981-126-333-0 (hardcover)
ISBN 978-981-126-419-1 (paperback)
ISBN 978-981-126-334-7 (ebook for institutions)
ISBN 978-981-126-335-4 (ebook for individuals)

For any available supplementary material, please visit
https://www.worldscientific.com/worldscibooks/10.1142/13055#t=suppl

This book presents the curious pathway that led me first to medicine. It also tells how I left practice for research, and where did teaching fit in. This could be useful to many students — high school, undergraduate, and even medical students — or beginning doctors, wondering about practice, research or teaching in these times of fantastic scientific advances? Many parents and grandparents, especially mothers, want their children to be doctors. Their children, at school, college, or university, wonder how to go about it.

This book is not about being a doctor. It is about the complexities of the pathway.

Students are often unaware of the twists and turns of careers. Many careers are available. Most will become practitioners. Many will become investigators. Some will combine teaching, research and practice. How are these choices made? This book introduces students to some of the ways that these choices arise. They are not as simple as one might think. They involve understanding how research, teaching and practice occur, and the influences that each can have on the others. They also show how curious the pathway to medicine can be.

This is not a handbook about how to become a doctor. It is about the complex pathways to the becoming. As you are, so was I a science student in school — then a university undergraduate interested in the sciences, next a clinical student moving onward to medical practice. But there were further paths. After practice, I became a professor questioning ideas (researching), exciting students (teaching), and applying methods (from the breadth of the humanities and arts, as well as the sciences: biology, mathematics, engineering and medicine). Now, fascinated by the questions students ask, I am challenging 'how it all works'.

Though the story begins gently, it leads more deeply into the relationships between teaching, research and practice, and their interactions. And it leads fiercely into challenging institutions, disciplines, governments and society.

I want you, students, to know these things, to be prepared for them, and to enjoy your careers as much as I have mine. But I also want you to recognize the damages that are occurring to science and medicine (and especially in the West). And I want you to be prepared to participate in repairing the damages, into taking the next steps.

"It is important that students bring a certain ragamuffin,
barefoot irreverence to their studies.
They are not here to worship what is known,
but to question it."
(Bronowski, 1975, modified)

"In science [and medicine] one must search for ideas.
If there are no ideas, then there is no science
[and no medicine].
Facts are not valuable when they conceal ideas.
Facts without ideas clutter up the mind and the memory."
(Belinski, 1811–1848, reported 1948, modified)

Chandrasekhar said:
"There were only two students in that graduate class ..."
Unable to contain himself, one hot-shot young dean
jumped up and almost shouted:
"That's it; that's the size of class that should be cancelled!"
Chandra completed his sentence:
"... and their names were Yang and Li."

For my wife Eleanor, and our sons, Hugh and Guy.
I was a studious Medical Student: I married the
Medical Librarian.
Eleanor (as figured by Don Bachardy, loving partner
of Christopher Isherwood) has been in my work
and life for more years than we can count;
together we have crossed five continents and
enjoyed many lives.

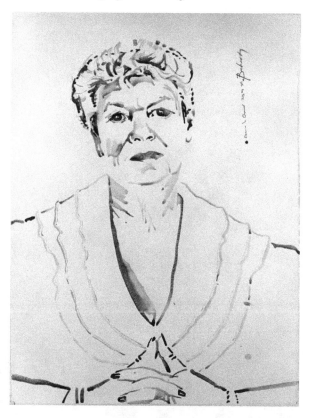

And to the memory of
Solly Zuckerman, Eric Ashton, Peter Lisowski, Alec Cave,
Tom Spence, John Young, and Len Freedman;
first teachers, then colleagues, then friends.

Acknowledgements

I am grateful to many teachers, mentors, colleagues and students who, over the years, have helped me as a physician and scientist.

I am especially indebted to Solly Zuckerman, Peter Lisowski, Eric Ashton, Alec Cave, Tom Spence, John Young, and Len Freedman, all of whom are now gone. I am also indebted to Neville Bruce, Fred Bookstein, Robin Crompton, Daniel Franklin, Rebecca German, Jens Hirschberg, Nina Jablonski, Robert Kidd, Algis Kuliukas, Paul O'Higgins, Ruliang Pan and Ken Wessen. And I thank my many other colleagues and students over the years (named throughout). They helped me with my work; I helped them with their work. Mostly we shared work together.

Scientific artists, artistic students, laboratory technicians, administrative assistants and many secretaries over the years have all helped with aspects of the materials on which this book is based. Artists have especially included Bill Pardoe from Birmingham, Joan Hives from Chicago, Erika Oller from Los Angeles, and Martin Thompson, Rebecca Davies and Sue Hayes from Western Australia.

I thank the four universities and medical schools in which I have worked. In spite of my 'diatribes' on occasion about educational institutions, they have all supported me most strongly.

I am also especially indebted to an incredible pattern of research funding during my life.

From 1961 to 1966, I received over £1 million in research funding from the Agricultural Research Council, UK, and the US

Public Health Service (awarded while I was in the UK). From 1966 to 1987, while in the USA, I received a total of US$4 million from the US Public Health Service and National Science Foundation, and from the Universities of Chicago and Southern California. From 1987 to 1997, in Australia, I received a total of A$3 million from the Australian Research Council, the National Health and Medical Research Council, the Medical Health and Research Foundation of Western Australia, the Raine Foundation, the Viertel Foundation, the CSIRO Australia, and the University of Western Australia.

Since 1997, I have continued to receive, unexpectedly, research funds as Emeritus Professor and Senior Honorary Research Fellow at UWA. These have included A$2.4 million from Australian sources (ARC, NHMRC, MHRFWA), and £2.7 million from UK sources (Leverhulme Trust Professorship, Leverhulme Research Grant, BBSRC Research Grants, Marie Curie Research Grant, and PALAEO and EVAN Research Grants [through University College London, University of Liverpool, and Universities of York and Hull], many of these jointly with research colleagues).

And finally, I have consistently been continually supported by my universities: all loyal to me. And this, especially, has engendered in me a reverse loyalty to my institutions.

People have always been most important; four have been with me much of the way.

The first was Tom Spence, who died in 1977. He started as a Junior Technician in Anatomy in Birmingham, but made the transition — extremely difficult at that time in the UK — to academic ranks, eventually retiring as Senior Lecturer! I continued to visit him over the years after my moves abroad. I remember so much our hours of discussion, and the teas (and for me a beer) supplied by his wife Joan to keep us going. The university required him to pass an examination to move from a technical to academic position. This drew me to help him with a year of essays and seminars in human and vertebrate anatomy. As a result, of course, this helped me broaden my anatomical knowledge far beyond just humans!

The second was Professor Peter Lisowski, whom I knew through Birmingham and, as he moved, Haile Selassie University, Ethiopia, University of Hong Kong, and finally University of Tasmania. Peter and I taught together, examined together, published together, and travelled together. Peter was the academic anvil upon which my ideas of the scientific bases of medicine were hammered out. Though we were both old-fashioned medical anatomists by training, we both had ideas that were over and beyond the traditional teaching of medical anatomy. Eleanor and I were grateful to be with him and Ei Yoke, his wife, only a few days before he died.

The third was Len Freedman, who spent many years at the University of Western Australia changing the original medical anatomy into the (then) new idea of human biology as the science underlying the human condition. I had first met Len at the University of Wisconsin during my Chicago days. But it was in Western Australia, with the total support of his then professor, David Allbrook, and of Neville Bruce and the other academic staff at UWA, that he elaborated these ideas and carried them back into the high schools and forward into the university, much more widely than just medical anatomy. Accordingly, then, when I arrived at UWA many years later, I found a human biology niche already created, and which I further supported. I have been with Len ever since, including his years in active retirement. In 2014, aged 90, he died a true academic's death: sitting up in bed with the light on, his glasses on his nose, and a book on his breast.

The final individuals, are, of course, my wife, Eleanor, and our sons, Hugh and Guy. Since 1954, when I first knew Eleanor, she has supported me and my work. She was originally a medical librarian. I was the kind of medical student who spent much time in the library (I could reach her the books on the top shelf!). Much more so, however, we helped each other in both our work and our lives, through our various migrations across the world. Sometimes the moves were initially tough, especially for her, but she fell in with them, made her own way, and remained indispensable to our work and life together. Even now we continue to travel the world (coronavirus permitting) for family, collegial, and research purposes.

Our sons, Hugh and Guy, though never likely to enter medicine, both participated in my work at different times. I remember Hugh, dissecting monkey feet for me as a slightly appalled teenager, and Guy, much more recently, making sure I knew who this book was for.

It has been a wonderful thing to write. Everything is so different now from the days when we first started nearly seventy years ago. Eleanor and I sometimes wish we were back at the beginning of it all and not near the end! But being near the end, we hope to influence some of you, the next generations, to make changes for yourselves, and for even later generations.

I especially thank World Scientific and its Editorial teams. Over the years, you have all worked on many of my books and edited volumes. It has been an especial pleasure to be with you on this, my latest, but not my last.

Charles Oxnard
Emeritus Professor and Honorary Senior Research Fellow
University of Western Australia

Contents

Part 1

You (Our Students) Must be Center Stage

Chapter 1

Chapter 1: You (Our Students) Must be Center Stage

Chapter 1

You (Our Students) Must be Center Stage

First, I was a doctor who treated patients. Later, I became a professor, questioning ideas (researching), exciting students (teaching), borrowing techniques (from the breadth of biology, bio-mathematics, and bio-medical engineering, as well as medicine), and challenging 'how it all works'. Then, I became the Last Established Professor (there will be no more!). Now I am a Senior Honorary Research Fellow and Professor Emeritus.

The First Established Professor had also given up medical practice. His 1989 autobiography, titled *Not a Proper Doctor*, was a delightful, albeit gentle, life story.

Yet his title leads to my question: "Aiming at Medicine?" Though also beginning gently, my question leads ferociously into how real teaching, research and practice interact, and how, ferociously, we must challenge ideas, colleagues, disciplines, institutions, governments and society.

> **I want knowledge of these ferocities to be useful**
> **To students, dreaming about futures**
> **To parents (especially doctors and scientists) wondering if**
> **students should now follow them**
> **To grandparents, always proud of grandchildren**
> **To anyone, interested in teaching, discovery,**
> **practice and service**
> **And to all, fearing today's regress, wanting**
> **tomorrow's progress.**

First: Three Students

A Medical Student in Birmingham, 1960

One student, near the end of my very first term of teaching in medical school at the University of Birmingham, UK, asked for an appointment to see me. That worried me! No student had ever made an appointment; I saw them every day in the anatomy dissecting lab!

"Do you remember what you said at the beginning of the course?"
She asked (there were very few women in medicine in those days!).
"What?"
I queried.
"Well, if we had any problems we were to feel free to talk with you about them."
"Yes!"
I said (with a sinking feeling).
"Well,"
she said,
(my sinking feeling deepened!)
"WELL,"
she repeated, stringing me along,
"WELL,"
she said again,
"I'M PREGNANT!"

You can imagine what ran through my mind! Don't forget, this was the early 1960s. The only ways I knew for procuring an abortion were many stiff gins, very long hot showers, horseback riding, falling downstairs, and a wire coat hanger!
"It's OK!"
she said, laughing at my obvious discomfort,
"OUR BABY IS VERY MUCH WANTED."

Most of the **dark things** that had bubbled up in my mind evaporated. We all celebrated.

But the real dark thing was that she left medicine!

A High School Student in Los Angeles, 1978

My secretary said that Nancy, an assistant in my outer office, wanted to know if she could talk to me. Of course, I agreed, so in she came (Nancy's family name was Figueroa and that says much in California). No one in her family had ever gone to University. But her teenage daughter, Julia, seemed very bright, and so she asked if I would talk with her. Of course, I agreed.

Julia came, and during our talk I showed her some of my own publications. At the end, when she was about to go, Julia asked if I would give her one of those papers.

"I'll do more than that,"
I said,
"I'll give you a whole book."

I gave her my then most recent book, **The Order of Man**. The feminists on campus had agreed to my using this title, the word **"man"** being the English translation of the word *homo*, the genus in the zoological *order* to which we belong. Julia asked me to write in it, so I did. I wrote:

"These are the Voyages of the Star Ship Julia,
*To Boldly Go where No Man **or Woman** has Gone Before."*

This was in the early days of Star Trek, long before they had their original, politically incorrect, statement: "Where No **Man** Has Gone Before."

Nowadays, a masculine Captain Kirk has mutated into female Captains as tough as Garrett, as ambitious as Shelby, as likeable as Jadzia, and as interestingly flawed as Janeway.

Years after, on a return visit to Southern California, I met Nancy again. She told me how much that talk had meant to Julia, that Julia still had the book, that she had indeed gone on to university (the first in her family), became qualified in pharmacy, and became a successful practitioner.

Wow! The wonders of teaching! Do we really know what our words may mean to students?

A Postgraduate Research and Teaching Student, 1990

In reviewing the status of a particular anatomy department, I had to interview, among others, a postgraduate research student who was also teaching anatomy to medical students. He was clearly absolutely fascinated by anatomy, outgoing to his students, deeply concerned with teaching as well as he could, and, I could see, a teacher very much liked. I asked during the interview:
"What about your research?"
He told me.

Later, at the kind of social occasion, that also occurs in such situations, I met him again over drinks. I repeated my question:
"Tell me more about your research in anatomy."
"Well,"
he said, honestly:
"To tell you the truth I am not very interested in my research. I do it because I know I have to publish for my career. I do it because it gives me something to tell people like you when you come around."
"So, why are you so interested in teaching anatomy?" I asked.

"Because I love the structure of human anatomy,"
he said,
"because I love the fact that it is so complete,"
"because I love to present this completed structure to the students,"
he continued,
"because there are no more questions to be asked!"

I have never forgotten his words. No matter how much this teacher is liked by his students, if he leaves them with the notion that his subject is complete, that there are no more questions to be asked, then I aver that he is a very bad teacher indeed.

It is my fervent desire that my students will always find that their own work raises new questions and challenges their own ideas. It is my fervent desire that my students will see how work in other disciplines can provide new questions for their own. It is even my fervent desire that my students in their various disciplines will provide new questions for other disciplines. It is my final fervent desire that new questions will always come thick and fast to my students.

Second: More Students

Later, in Los Angeles, when I was the Dean of the Graduate School, I also remained a Professor in the Medical School. I developed a special relationship with the medical student classes. Many of the students had started to realize that it might be important that they have a science side to their medical lives. Partly, this was because of medicine's increasing scientific base. Partly, it was because they could see that the pressures of practice might need to be leavened by research and teaching. Mostly, it was because medicine in the USA was a postgraduate degree — following on from various and varied undergraduate backgrounds.

First, I was approached by a group of medical students (leaders, medical students Julie Graylow and Hugh Allen) who wanted to do medical research. Would I help them start up a 'Medical Student Research Group'? I found them genuine research projects, not just bottle washing, in different labs around the medical school and hospitals. As many as twenty students participated each year. They were so much into research that many subsequently gave papers at the Western Medical Students Research Forum. All wanted additional 'research strings' to their 'practice bow'.

Next, I was approached by a student group whose undergraduate degrees were in engineering (led by medical student, and prior undergraduate engineer, Dan Zinder). They wanted to start an 'Engineers in Medicine Group' and wanted my support as their faculty director. I well remember taking them to a factory making artificial lenses for cataracts. The students (and I) were nonplussed to realize that the quality control in this factory involved rejection rates of more than 98%, so tight were the specifications.

Partly as a result of these endeavors, and partly because I had previously followed Joe Ceithaml as Director of the Chicago MD/PhD program, I became the first director of a new 'MD/PhD program' at USC. In those days, these were new developments in the US medical curriculum.

All these students could see the excitement of combining practice and research.

Third: Some 'Festering' Ideas

The above are just a few student stories among many in my academic life. But my aim in writing this book is not autobiographical.

No, my aim is to get off my chest a set of ideas about education and universities, about science and medicine, about teaching

*and research, about the way universities work, even about impli-
cations outside universities, but most of all about students and
professors.*

Despite having had a wonderful life in science and medicine, these *ideas* have 'festered' in my mind for many years. If they can be of any use to those hoping to do science, technology and medicine, to those wondering where to go next in universities (whatever their interests may be), or even to those just interested in what universities are, their functions in society, and how they are changing, then I will be happy.

One reads reports, often from education departments, teaching commissions, review bodies, governmental committees, and others, about what is needed for teachers 'to lift their game', for it is often assumed that the problems are teachers! We worry that educational standards (in our kindergartens, schools and colleges, not only universities) have greatly slipped in recent decades. And teachers are usually blamed! This is at the same time that education is on the up in so many countries (especially in the East). These critical reports often suggest improvements: strategic plans, performance indicators, learning walks, flipped classrooms, MOOCS, teaching instructors, annual reviews, educational questionnaires, complex timesheets, even, now, on-line teaching replacing face-to-face learning, or any of the other flotsam and jetsam infecting teaching at almost every level.

Often, such reports come up with recommendations to reject what manifestly works, such as rejection of phonics, rejection of mathematics, rejection of lectures, seminars, and small classes, and very especially rejection of one-on-one teaching, even rejection of literacy and numeracy (mangled through messaging by, now, generations of 'eye-pad' and 'eye-phone' users). The whole thing is clear. Student outcomes are best when teaching is mostly teaching-led, rather than student-led. In reading, phonics-based instruction works and should not be replaced by look-and-guess. In maths, problem-solving with understanding works, and should be implemented and non-negotiable. And so too, all this applies at university level.

Very often such reports come up with one or a very few recommendations that, it is alleged, are the solution. They always include: *doing more with less!* And: *fixing one thing, will fix all!* Such notions seem not to recognize that doing more with less, or fixing just one or perhaps two points, are highly unlikely to do any good. They seem never to understand that the true problem is multidimensional; it needs many changes taken together.

It never seems to register that what might really help would be, *concurrently*:

better: salaries, careers, and support,
reduced: testing and questionnaires, administrative interferences, and students per staff,
recognizing: not only the teaching-research nexus that worked in the past, but even the teaching-research-practice triad in the profession of medicine, so important now and even more so next.

It never seems to register that a career structure is needed wherein *career development* occurs by recognizing the fun of teaching and telling new stories, and that this, in turn, stems from the excitement of research and tackling new questions.

All this contrasts with the present, where it seems as if *career development* can only be achieved:
by changing from teaching and research to management,
by moving from classroom and laboratory to office,
and even, as so frequently happens:

by leaving education completely for a 'proper' career-progressive profession!

As I was working on these thoughts, I came across Gabbie Stroud's *Teacher*. What a wonderful book!

Gabbie Stroud: School Teacher

Gabbie's book is about primary-school teaching and is:

> *"An achingly heartfelt reflection on how bureaucracy dehumanises teachers and children.*
> *How the joys of teaching and learning are turning into despair.*
> *How children are becoming less important than outcomes."*
>
> *"Gabbie's story needs to be shouted from the roof-tops.*
> *She very elegantly shows us why and how schools have to change.*
> *'Teacher' made me both laugh and cry. I loved it!"*

Until that moment I had not known Gabbie's primary-school story: about her classrooms, playgrounds and outings. But I immediately realized that her primary-school story applies equally to my medical-school story: about my seminar rooms, laboratories and clinics.

Almost point by point, what Gabbie describes for schools is occurring also in universities and hospitals. Because it is so long since we had our own children, this had escaped Eleanor and I.

Earlier, my students became doctors, specialists, and professors. Quite a number have now retired, and some have even, regrettably, died (I am older than you think)!

Now, many of my recent students, in spite of being among my best in over sixty years (two followed me to Australia from London, one won a double doctorate, four got doctorates with honours [not easy!], some published in *Nature* and the *Proceedings of the Royal Society*, three were national prize winners, several became journal editors, one became president of an academic society, many have become medical consultants), have also included *ten excellent students who have gone away because there is no university career for them in Australia!*

When I was young, doctors (usually men) were often (and sometimes overly) keen to encourage their children (usually boys) to follow them into medicine.

Those doctors, many of my generation, are now retiring early (we were trained to be doctors but have become accountants, administrators, and assessors) and often warn their grandchildren, both girls and boys, against it. This book is partly about this, and why it is a 'bad thing'.

Of course, medicine has changed over the years. It would be curious if it were not so.

Time was: and the art of medicine increasingly included the science of medicine, or evidence-based medicine ('evidence-based' is a forbidden term in Trump's White House Media!).
Time is: and medicine (and its science) is becoming defensive-based, lawyer-proofed, and grievance-resistant.
Time may be: and the medical and health professions may become totally subordinated to political control, bureaucratic distrust, and the imperatives of management and profit.

Ancestors to Teaching and Research!

This book is also about *thoughts* that have *evolved* over many years. And to a doctor who is also an evolutionary biologist, if *thoughts* have *evolved*, they therefore have *ancestors*, many *ancestors*!

"It is important that students bring a certain ragamuffin, barefoot irreverence to their studies; they are not here to worship what is known, but to question it."

(Bronowski, 1975, modified).

As a beginning teacher at the University of Birmingham, UK, with two others, Heather Beaumont and Terry Baker, we often discussed how better to teach our medical students.

Partly this was because we were new to the task. We did not want to just present a set of facts to be memorized. We wanted understanding, not memory, to be the watchword. We didn't care too much if a student could not bring a scientific term or medical name to mind. We did care that they knew what it was, how it worked, and what happened when it failed.

We also decided that the separate bits we each had to teach should be integrated. We did not want our own parts of our discipline (in those days, anatomy, histology and embryology, all parts of today's human biology) to be seen as separate. We also did not want our overall discipline, human biology, to be thought of as separate from the rest of medicine. Even then, we were aware of the *isolated and isolating towers* within academia and the professions!

We wanted our students to know that it is through obtaining new knowledge and through researching that teaching and learning are leavened and live. We wanted them to understand the nature of the bipartite nexus of research and teaching.

And finally, as well as being a physician, I wanted the students to understand that the professionalism of medicine requires a tripartite nexus: teaching, research and practice. True practice is not just practice alone!

It was somewhat unusual in those days for relatively junior individuals, such as we were, to be allowed to change teaching, rather than simply following an older teaching pattern from an older generation. Of course, all we could change were our own minor contributions to our little group of twelve medical students. But how *good* it was that three young teachers could be allowed to integrate our different parts of the discipline; how *good* it was that those twelve students were able to discuss and question with us; and how *good* it was that our student-to-staff ratio was 4:1. These three *'goods'* are among the bases for the finest learning and teaching.

Our teaching was never 'evaluated', never 'questionnaired', and certainly never 'bureaucratized'! We were just *trusted* to get on with the job. We *gloried* in our students' excellent results. We worked so *enthusiastically* for those students, who all wanted to do well. They worked *incredibly hard* for us. Many became *lifelong* friends!

> *"In science [and medicine] one must search for ideas.*
> *If there are no ideas, then there is no science [and no medicine].*
> *Facts are not valuable when they conceal ideas.*
> *Facts without ideas clutter up the mind and the memory."*
> (Belinski [1811–1848] reported in 1948, here slightly modified).

> And also:
> *"Facts are chiels that winna ding, an' downa be disputed".*
> (Burns, 1759–1796).

What happened to us in teaching also happened in research. In Solly Zuckerman's department in Birmingham at that time, as young researchers, we were thrown in at the deep end. Lifelines were available if we started to flounder, but the research atmosphere in that department was so exciting — there was so much discussion and questioning among us all; everyone was so interested in what everyone else was doing — that lifelines were rarely needed. Coffee time was a time for swapping science; very exciting science indeed!

> *"To live for a time close to great minds is the very*
> *best form of education."*
>
> (John Buchan, 1940).

Coffee time had not degenerated into what it so often is today: groans about impossible administrative requirements and teaching loads, about little or no research funding, about few or no jobs, and about major, major job insecurity!

In effect, then, in both teaching and research, we three young academics felt bonded to each other — to the exciting minds with whom we worked, to the living department in which we were located, to the medical school as a whole, and even to the whole university.

Even though we were, of course, all 'just' employees, and the university 'just' our employer, we felt we had more than 'just' an employee-employer relationship. We felt we had stakes in our students, colleagues and professors, and in our institutions, disciplines and professions, that were so much greater than being merely in employment.

We wanted to 'give' to our students, colleagues, professors, institutions, disciplines and professions, in ways far beyond those 'given' by employees to employers. We felt a sense of deep loyalty and trust.

And we believed that our disciplines, our universities, our professions, our professors, our colleagues, and our students would, in turn, 'give' to us. It turned out that it was so: there was incredible reciprocal loyalty and trust!

And this did not occur just at the University of Birmingham. For many years after Birmingham (at the Universities of Chicago, Southern California, and Western Australia), I continued to have such feelings in spades.

It was only many years later still, luckily for me only during my so-called 'retirement', that such feelings would fade, that we would gradually become 'just employees' in thrall to 'employers', that the 'collegial academy' would gradually die, being replaced by a 'business house', with a 'commercial ethos', run by 'managers'. Managers would decide what we should do, how we should be judged, and even if we should continue to be employed! Trust, loyalty, help and security were to gradually disappear. How things have changed!

Beginnings, Endings, and 'In-between-ings'

I have almost always been involved in students' beginnings and endings. At the University of Chicago, as Dean of the College (of Letters, Arts and Sciences), I had to welcome the incoming students and congratulate the outgoing ones.

I well remember a talk to the Chicago 'freshers' and their parents that I concluded with:

"With this welcome comes a parting. Now, students go one way, parents another!" — words which, to be honest, I had 'borrowed' from the previous Dean and Physicist, Professor Roger Hildebrand. I found that I had a lot of parents in the front rows, quietly crying! In contrast, the students were raring to get on 'their' way!

Perhaps the Chicago talk I most enjoyed was a degree day offering that I had entitled 'The Curmudgeon Correspondence: Letters from an Old Don to a Young Professor'. These were a series of letters that I had (supposedly) found in the University Archives. They were patterned, of course, upon C. S. Lewis's *The Screwtape Letters*.

On such an occasion, at Chicago, one was supposed to speak (on orders from President Levi) for only twelve minutes! (One colleague twitted the President by entitling his talk 'Twelve Minutes and the Glory of God'). For my talk, I 'found' about a dozen 'Curmudgeon Letters'. The letters had instructions from an old Don, Curmudgeon, to a young Professor, Bilbo, on how to 'fail' the students! They had themes truly pertinent to the students of those days, for example: 'The Law of Undulation' (what goes around comes around), 'The Principle of the False Dichotomy' (using simplicity to hide complexity), and especially 'Science for the People' (something much in the minds of the nuclear protesters of those days of the 1960s). I was therefore able to give four talks of 12 minutes' worth of letters, varying the mix of 'letters' at each of the degree day 'sittings'.

Edward Levi was so pleased. He said it was the first time he had not had to listen to the same speech four times!

Later still, at the University of Southern California, I talked to the graduating doctorates each year. The university was so big that, after the President had 'blessed' all 10,000 or so students with a doff of his cap, they then split into their discipline groups to actually receive their diplomas. As I was Dean of the Graduate School, my satellite ceremonies were for much smaller numbers of PhD recipients. Again, therefore, I had chances to philosophize about academia and the wider world.

One year I had a very tall student (well over 6 feet, Figure 1.1).

Edward was really in the School of Public Administration, but because he was doing a PhD, he came under my aegis.

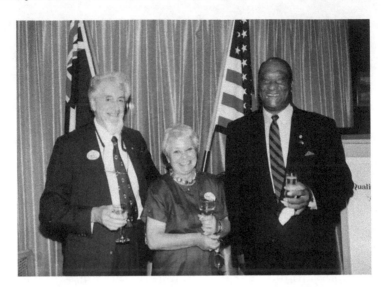

Figure 1.1:   Edward Perkins, the US Ambassador to Australia years later, and Eleanor and I at the US Consulate in Perth.

We were both amazed when we met in Perth, many years later, with him, Edward Perkins, as the US Ambassador, and Eleanor an employee of the State Department, in the US Consulate in Perth.

One year I was invited to give the degree day speech to the Southern California medical class. The speaker, chosen by the students, was required to be from outside the university. The students that year were smart. While I was still technically in Southern Cal, when the students requested the administration to invite me to give the speech, they knew that Eleanor and I were about to move to Australia. On their degree day, we would actually be '*just* out-side the university'. So, we were both brought back from Australia that first year away!

Because of this, I knew all the students (Eleanor too, because some of them had been in our home!). We also knew their parents because, four years before, we had welcomed those parents at the beginning of their medical students' careers. I was able to share insider thoughts about learning that were recognized by both students and parents, even to the point of asking them questions — 'real' ones — during the talk. The students roared with approval. They were well aware of my habit of asking 'real questions' of 'real individuals' in lectures, and hoping for 'real answers'!

Later still, in a graduation talk at the University of Western Australia, I again pontificated about teaching and research; about questioning and challenging; about universities and academia, an ancestor to this book!

Each of these occasions was a time for reflection on what we, in education, are about.

> *"The greatest event in the world today is [...] the advent of a new way of living, due to science [and medicine], a change in the conditions of work and the structure of society which began not so very long ago in the West, and is now reaching out over all mankind."*
>
> Not written today, but by Vannevar Bush a long time ago!

And there have been many *in-between* occasions when I was asked to talk, over and beyond the usual teaching, research, and clinical lectures and seminars.

At the University of Southern California, for example, I was asked by Dean Joan (at one time the Dean of Women!) to support an Undergraduate Student Honours Society called 'Mortar Board'. Would I give them regular talks? I did, and I even wrote them up as a series of short essays and gave them to the Mortar Board students to criticize, with the thought that they might appear someday as a book. The students were delighted to be included in the writing process. We had some great discussions, but it never did appear as a book, except in some of the ideas in this book; and this is forty years later.

As a result, I was elected to Phi Gamma Delta (button hole: a golden rose). This is a *graduate women's honor society* (and they didn't change the pronouns in my pledge)!

A somewhat similar invitation came at the University of Western Australia. As the first Head of the Division of Science and Agriculture (read today as Executive Dean), I was asked to give an academic year's worth of half-hour discussions each week with Inge Rigby, a host on the local University Wireless Station. (Wireless eventually became radio, and anyway the University Radio Station, like the University Press, is now defunct [though I understand the press now is being revived in a new format]). Inge wanted the thoughts of a new academic (new to UWA at least) on universities and academia, research and teaching, students and staff, governments and funding, and so on.

I was so nervous on that first occasion that I grossly over-prepared. But I quickly realized that, if I was going to give one every week for two semesters, I would not have time for that. So, I subsequently did them 'al fresco', and they were much better for it. They also owed much to Inge Rigby's acute questioning. The series had the jaded title of 'Beyond the Ivory Tower', but I could not get Inge to change it! Again, those talks became a preliminary to this book.

I also met Jane Figgis who ran *Science Bookshop* for the ABC in Perth. She asked me to review Chandrasekhar's beautiful book, *Truth and Beauty: Aesthetics and Motivations in Science*. I was especially pleased to do a half hour review of this book for 'Steam Radio' because, of course, I had known 'Chandra' in Chicago. He was a delightful, very quiet Indian, the Morton D. Hull Distinguished Professor in Astronomy and Astrophysics. I have an anecdote about him that is absolutely pertinent to the thesis of this book.

Thus, there used to be 'All Deans' meetings of the Midwest 'Big Ten Universities'. Actually, the grouping was indeed the ten large state universities in the Midwest, but it also further included two small but excellent private institutions, Northwestern University and The University of Chicago. There was a year when the Chicago Science Dean (who was, as it happens, an Australian) was unable to go to the Deans' meeting, so he deputized Chandra to go in his place. The main matter for discussion was the question: how small should a class be before, in the interest of educational efficiency(!), it should be cancelled? Perhaps twelve for an undergraduate class, perhaps eight for a graduate class?

There was much discussion but Chandra, so quiet and gentle, did not participate. At the end of the meeting, it was customary for the Chairman to go clockwise around the room asking what was Illinois' opinion, what was Wisconsin's opinion, and so on. It happened that Chandra was just on his right and therefore the last one to speak.

What was Chicago's opinion? Chandra spoke. He told the story of how he had forgotten that he had a graduate seminar on Saturday mornings in a quarter when he was on sabbatical at the Yerkes Observatory in Wisconsin. In order to meet with his graduate class, he had to drive down to Chicago every Friday night to give the seminar on Saturday morning, and then drive back to his Yerkes sabbatical.

"There were only two students in the class ..."

Unable to contain himself one hotshot young dean jumped up and almost shouted:

"That's it; that's the sort of class that should be cancelled!"

Chandra completed his sentence:

"... and their names were Yang and Li!" (Both subsequently got Nobel Prizes.)

The Wider Academy in the West

When, eventually in 1997, I retired, I thought that, in retirement, I ought to contribute to the discussion about the problems of university education.

But no! I quickly found that my research and teaching were to enter yet another growth phase, to continue unabated. This was because my research funding continued, my teaching was what I wanted to offer, and my administrative responsibilities became zero!

The university still gives me an office, a staff number, an academic title, an address from which to publish and receive grants, and travel insurance *gratis* (and for my wife!) when we travel on university business! As a result, in retirement, I have published more papers and books, done more research, obtained more grant money, and have more graduate students and postdocs than, perhaps, at any other time in my life. There has, thus, been little time for that broader contribution.

However, education in Australia, and indeed the world, is changing. For a long time now, universities have been described as getting better, but have actually been getting worse. A number of British universities think they are getting better because they are getting closer to Oxford and Cambridge. I fact, in my opinion, all are getting worse, but Oxford and Cambridge are getting worse more quickly, drawing down closer to the others!

Almost everywhere there are more students but fewer teachers, more administration but less research, more institutions but much less money. This had so hurt the universities that they had to take many more (money-carrying) overseas students. This policy, forced by government reductions, is now further worsened by the combination of Covid-19 lockdowns and China's economic policies. It has resulted not only in major financial losses, but also in the even more serious loss of the cultural elements that they bring to us, and the parts of our cultures they take home.

The USA, with its highly plural higher education system, has escaped some of these losses. In the USA, the broad mix of universities — the elite privates (like Harvard), the even more elite (as they would have it) private colleges (like Williams), the usually private, religious institutions (some very good indeed), the top public state universities (also excellent), the excellent land grant universities (as they originally were), the intermediate-level state institutions, the public city and local community institutions, and a wide range of others — all form a very complex system not paralleled in any other country.

The funding of that system is equally complex: federal, state, city, land grant, many religious contributors, the large and complex range of private foundations and other charitable groups, individual giving by alumni (on a scale so different from that in any other country), private individual giving (by people such as Bill and Melinda Gates who want to make a 'difference'), and incredibly generous business and industrial funding. These supports are far greater than those in any other country (but see China later!).

Indeed, the endowments of several single US universities, alone, are greater than the total funds of all of education at all levels in Australia!

As a result of this complexity, it is generally difficult to 'screw' the entire US system at once.

In contrast, in most other OECD countries, including Australia, governments are the mainstay of universities. And they are becoming increasingly poorer mainstays. All universities have suffered. This has especially happened in Australia where public funding (in constant dollars) of universities is about one third of what it was when I first came here (1987).

University funding in Australia may be yet further decreased in order to allow increased funding of high schools! How silly, to reduce the resources for university places for school leavers just as places for school entrants are being increased!

There seems to be no understanding that increasing one arena of a linked system requires increasing all others in the system because, by definition, it is a flow chart. One is reminded of the good value of a 'head start' for Chicago preschoolers in the 1960s. But damage followed when these students moved into grade school and: *the support was not continued at that new level!*

During my retirement, all this seemed such a disaster that I felt I could not make a dent in such a tsunami of change. *So, I did not take on that challenge!* I probably saved myself a lot of heartache. *But perhaps I made a major mistake.* Perhaps I should have thrown myself on the pyre. The smoke might just have been white; it might just have helped!

Teaching and Research in the East

These damages to many western educational systems have not occurred in many of the countries in the East. Of course, their systems generally started from a much lower base and that made it easy to move up.

China, for example, had to start from ground zero after total closing of the universities and the loss of entire generations of academics resulted from Mao's Cultural Revolution. I was in China as a guest of the China Medical Board every second year following that time. In addition to being invited to give research presentations in my small research area, I helped Chinese colleagues to restart their careers and their disciplines.

Of course, the first thing they had to do was get the teaching going; that took the first years after Mao's *university-killing* Cultural Revolution.

It was wonderful how quickly it all occurred. I saw one-year 'bare-foot doctor' medical schools on my first visit, two-year medical schools on my second visit only two years later, and so on to four-year medical schools only a few years after that. Incredible effort! We further helped by sending them all our secondhand textbooks. The growth of these medical schools in size, complexity and quality in such a short time was amazing. Of course, the nature of government in China is such that this could be mandated. At first copying, but later improving upon, the great universities of the USA, Germany, the UK, and now beating many of them, the top Chinese institutions are now making major advances in their own right!

After teaching, China next tackled the question of getting research going, because there was a clear understanding by the Communist Party that communicating knowledge without also adding to knowledge is sterile. It was in this phase that I was especially involved.

On my first visit (1980), they wanted me to talk about the uses of computers in increasing our understanding of anatomy. I did this, and they were very excited; but of course, they had no computers!

Two years later, local Chinese colleagues gave two papers using computer techniques. They were not good papers, but at least they were doing it. Two years later still there was a small session of papers using computational methods; some of them were good! This was a fantastic rate of change, mandated and supported of course, and unmatcheable in the West!

Let us now jump quickly to today. From such a beginning, China has totally taken to computers as we all know. But do we all know that China has been so successful that China-based super-computers (Sunway TaihuLight, and Tianhe-2) have leapfrogged all rivals to be named the world's most powerful systems by factors of nearly ×10 (as of December 2019)? Of course, one has to be careful; there are a number of different ways of measuring computer power!

Thus, the USA (with 108 supercomputers in 2018) no longer dominates the world. China (with 229) has overtaken the USA, Japan is third with 31, and the UK fourth with 20. Australia has just 5! But then we in Australia give the defence that we always give: we are too small for this league. But we also say that we 'punch above our weight'. I wonder, do we really?

Most recently of all, an Australian woman has been lauded, rightly so, for being in the vanguard of quantum computing. Though it does not yet do much, quantum computing has great promise for the near future. Are we aware that China is well ahead in this area? Are we aware enough that China's expertises in these new cybernetic systems parallel her current decades and more of other developments on land, sea, air, cloud and space?

Today, huge spending is being thrown around in China: trillions of yuan on all things scientifico-technical-medical. Does China want to achieve knowledge dominance? Over the next few years, national plans include injecting more than 3.5 trillion yuan (more than A$10 trillion) into this arena. Of course, Australia cannot be in such a league, but I submit that the West as a whole is not in this league. In the West, science and technology just do not count to that degree to government!

During these early China visits, I also did one or two very small things.

"Will you please read anatomical words into a tape recorder?"

my Chinese colleagues asked,

"We don't know how to pronounce them."

So, I did. I would spend perhaps two hours in each medical college reading the words. As a result, there may be a generation of medics in China who pronounce anatomical terms with a 'North Country English' accent. The word 'malleolus' is pronounced 'malÃy-uh-les' in Oxford and Cambridge, but 'Mally-Oh-L-Us' in the North of England!

I even helped them to make applications for jobs abroad.

"What is this thing called a CV (curriculum vitae) that we need to have to go abroad?"

they asked,

"We don't have them."

And it was true; certainly, they were not producing teaching text-books nor research papers; no 'journals' in the Western sense in China at that time. So, I quizzed them.

"You teach?"

I asked; they agreed.

"You have written materials about your teaching; they are the equivalent of a teaching portfolio!".

"You do research?"

I queried; they agreed.

"You write reports about it; they are the equivalent of research publications in the West!"

"Yes."

And so, I helped them to prepare CVs to go abroad. (Later, I was, myself, the recipient of some of these researchers into Australia.)

Also in those China visits in the 1980s and 1990s (and funded by the China Medical Board), I was invited to discuss with Chinese colleagues the kinds of research (in my general area of expertise) that they might do. I agreed to try.

"We are interested in human development," they said, "but we do not yet have the technology, the electron microscope and so on, to look at the sperm, the egg and the early embryo. Is there some other part of human development we could study at this time?"

"Well," I said, "you could look at later stages of development. That needs only the light microscope."

(These later stages were starting to be somewhat less interesting to Western embryology [as it was at that time] because of extreme interest in the electron microscope and the very earliest stages of development.)

"There is still a lot to find with the light microscope."

But of course, I also said, "Such research would need to be statistically based with reasonable samples."

"How many specimens in a sample?"

they asked.

"Well, most statisticians would want perhaps sixteen or even sixty, but I, as a biologist, am willing to try with even just six!"

"Oh, we could manage that!"

came the confident answer.

And later that visit, she showed me a museum of pots with many hundreds of specimens at different ages following conception:

three months, four months, five months … eight months,
nine months, ten months …
eleven months, twelve months, thirteen months!

This was the beginnings of the 'One Child Policy' with not only the inevitable 'embryocides' and 'foeticides', but also 'infanticides'. Most appeared normal as far as I could see!

There is the story (I hope apocryphal) of the nurse who had to give lethal injections to 'extra' (unwanted) babies. She injected one of a twin pair, but then, upon being told she had injected the wrong one, promptly turned around and injected the other!

Of course, at that point (early 1980s) I knew nothing about the One Child Policy. But on those scientific occasions, usually held in one or other of the sacred mountains, one would walk on mountain paths, two by two, with a Chinese colleague. One such meeting was at Omei San, another at Lu San ('san' meaning mountain, the same character as 'yama' as in Fuji-Yama — Mount Fuji!). Walking two-by-two in the mountains is when people say what is in their hearts. One Chinese colleague was so upset at these policies — but could do nothing!

I wondered, should I talk to the US State Department when I got home? Then I came to my senses. I was not the only American visitor in China. Far more senior Americans had been there before me. The US Government obviously knew about it but was keeping quiet!

To return to improvements in teaching and research, they have happened not only in China. India, Thailand, Indonesia, South Korea, Singapore, Hong Kong (as it was then) and other Asian countries have all long realized the value of strengthening their educational systems.

Of course, these societies have an advantage that we of the West lack. They are all societies that respect — even revere — age, thinking, wisdom, teaching, learning, and the individuals so involved. Western societal customs, prejudiced views of age, the low status of teachers and researchers, and the reductions of funds for schools and universities are all so negative. Indeed, in Australia, the word 'academic' is very often pejorative!

China knew the opposite very early!

"We must catch up with this advanced level of world science ...
either in peaceful competition ...
or in any aggressive war ...
which the enemy may unleash."

(Zhou Enlai, Report on the **Question of the Intellectuals, 1956**)

We need to take heed of Zhou Enlai!

Further Thoughts Today

Most recently of all, further reflections have been forced upon me. The UK gave me my degrees and my academic start.

But it was in the USA that I had my main career. It was in the USA that I became a Full Professor. It was in the USA that I was first elected to fellowships of scientific bodies, presidents of academic societies, and deans in universities.

Latterly, Australia has also been good to me. Australia has given me an excellent final ten-year career, and after that, an incredible twenty-five years (so far) of active retirement. I have had the unique gift of ten Australian Research Council grants in my retirement alone.

Even more remarkably, however, the UK and USA have also continued to help me in my supposed retirement. The UK has supported me through the Leverhulme Trust, the Novartis Foundation, BBSRC grants, and Marie Curie and Paleo Actions. The USA likewise has helped me through awards from the American Associations of Anatomy, of Physical Anthropology, and of Human Biology.

Finally, however, Australia has supported me in a new way in retirement. In 2013, I was 'dobbed in' by a colleague (Professor Miranda Grounds, with the collusion of Jane Figgis) to give a series of popular lectures to the Mature Adult Learning Association (MALA). The aim is to help older adults, mainly retired professionals, who are looking to learn new things. MALA had many classes on topics such as art, history, and languages, but almost nothing on science and medicine.

So, with the help of Hazel Butorac and her late husband Joe (both of MALA), I offered, in 2014, a ten-lecture course titled 'Science and Medicine, on Four Continents, and over Sixty Years'. I have continued to do this, with ten to twenty new lectures every year, to the present time. Of course, the aim of MALA is to help older people keep *their* brains active. But whatever may be their desire, the effect of MALA has also been to keep *my* brain active. I have enjoyed working with MALA and its mature, thinking, and questioning clientele enormously. And I even think that a course of such lectures might be useful for introducing university freshers to modern thinking in science and medicine. But this has not, so far, eventuated. The university has too many problems to take such an idea on board!

I am not grumbling! But I do wonder if such a series of talks might also increase high school and university students' interests in their futures. Anyway, such post-retirement experiences made me realize that these thoughts, leading to this book, were there. Perhaps I should have taken up the cudgels sooner!

Of course, there are other benefits. I recently had to undergo a bilateral inguinal herniorraphy. The surgeon was one of my old students, the anaesthetist another. I wondered, before I went under the knife, had I been nice to them? But then I remembered the words of the Hippocratic Oath (actually for me: The Declaration of Geneva):

> *"I will give to my teachers the respect and gratitude*
> *which are their due."*

They both did that, even remembering my jokes.

A Caveat

I must record that a considerable portion of this book is based not only upon written materials, but also upon several generations of computers, crackly audio tapes, poor video discs, ancient memory sticks, and most of all upon memories, often somewhat faded and often, too, partly incorrect. Everything is, no doubt, riddled with misinterpretation and 'misremembery'.

So, not everything I have written here is true. Though I have notes, many are almost indecipherable; though I have computer discs, they are outmoded; though I have memory sticks, most of them are for older versions of computers; though I have thoughts, many of them are fading fast; though I had many older colleagues who could have helped, most now are dead!

But I have younger colleagues, many originally my students; they continue to help. And I have a loyal wife, a medical librarian in a previous life; her librarian's 'organizationship' has brought order to the whole thing.

Part 2

How It Happened to Me (A Road Less Travelled)

Chapters 2–5

'A Road Less Travelled' examines the curious pathway that led me to medicine. It also tells how I left practice for research. And where did teaching fit? This road may be of interest to anyone thinking of entering practice, research or teaching, or (better) any two, or even (best) all three, in these times of fantastic advances.

Chapter 2: A Passion for Science and Medicine

Chapter 5: First Practice:
The Teaching/Research/Practice Triad

2 Chapter A Passion for Science and Medicine

"CCCRRRRRAAAAACK! Charles Oxnard had just hit himself on the head with a brick."

A small boy was trying to impress a small girl by throwing half-bricks into the air.

"He had forgotten that what goes up may come down. Then he tasted the liquid that ran down his face: salty."

The small girl could see it was red!

At that point, the small boy didn't know that the special structure of the scalp means that it easily bleeds.

"He had just discovered the Law of Gravity."

The words in quotes are words from an 'Essay for Teacher' entitled: *Charles Oxnard: A Passion for Science and Medicine*. It was written as a result of a half-way-across-the-world telephone interview conducted by my grandson, David. His essay concluded:

"Charles Oxnard is important to me because he gave me a microscope, and he is my grandpa! He truly has a fascinating career in science and medicine."

What David didn't know was that it was the blood running down my face that fascinated me (shades of Harvey), rather than the discovery of gravity (á la Newton).

These are a small grandson's words, and I am truly proud of them! He and his wife have now presented us with a first great granddaughter. Ingrid will receive the same first book, *Wombat*

Stew, that we gave David so many years ago! (None of our children are willing to give up their copies!)

The Start of the Passion

That passion may have started even earlier when my four-year-old sister developed rheumatic fever. I was so impressed by Dr. Kerr, who came to see her.

"You know, Mrs. Oxnard,"

he said to my mother, in his Scots brogue,

"it is wonderful. Years ago, these children all died; today they all live."

He was talking about the use of M and B (prontosil), the first sulphonamide available in the late 1930s, therefore predating penicillin (which did not become generally available for civilians until the end of the second world war).

Up to that point when, as a small boy, I was asked by adults:
"What do you want to be?"
I would answer: train driver, bus conductor, policeman, or some such, as one did at that age. But after Dr. Kerr's visit, I happened to answer:
"Doctor."
Ever after, my mother (who had been a nurse before she was married) would, when the question was asked, clap her hand over my mouth and say for me:
"He says he wants to be a doctor."
Of course, this is an early anecdote. The real stimuli came later, but some not very much later!

Before the second world war, my father took us from the North Country to Southampton where he worked on the Spitfire at Supermarine Works. During the phony war, the government decided that children should be evacuated to the country. Evacuations were based upon the schools. There was no way that my mother would allow that, so she took me out of school. (My sisters were not at risk; they had not yet started school.)

As a result, I missed the first year of schooling and did not re-enter school until we all moved to Scotland after the war started. I was therefore somewhat older than the other kids in that first class in Scotland. But at least I could read; in those days, one learnt to read at one's mother's knee!

That first Scottish teacher's job, therefore, was to teach me to write. She was a white-haired, superannuated, martinet of a teacher (Miss Kerr) who had been brought back into teaching because of the war. As I was left handed, when I held the slate pencil in my right hand, my knuckles were crunched up. She achieved her task by hitting me on the crunched knuckles with a ruler every time she passed me. I learnt to write with knuckles straight very quickly, and was immediately elevated to the next class (and away from her!).

The next class contained three classes in one room (because of the teacher shortage and it was in a small village school). That was serendipitous because that teacher (Miss Parrot) allowed me to do the work of all three classes as she moved over them.

Eventually I achieved Dr. Thompson's (the Head Master's) class. (He called himself *the Heid Yin*: I had no idea what that meant!)

A Primary School Head Master

One usually thinks first of the well-known people who have been responsible for one's career and one's life. Yet my first real stimulus came from the enthusiasm of that relatively unknown *Heid Yin* of that tiny primary school in Gullane, East Lothian, Scotland.

One day he told me that in our school the education was very classical. The subjects taught were English (mainly English grammar, taught the Scottish way; how useful that turned out to be for an academic career), geography (mainly Scottish geography; with the many times I drew the outline of Scotland, I could almost do it in my sleep), history (mainly Scottish history; when we did Bannockburn I was OK, but the day we did Flodden Field, as the only English boy in a Scottish School, was the day I had to run home; luckily I was long and thin and very fast), and mathematics (one could be stopped to do 'ten mental' anywhere in the school, even in the playground, and at any time of the day).

"But," he said, "there are other subjects that we do not teach. One of them is a thing called science." He may have seen that I was interested in his curio cabinet (displaying a kukri and kris, an ostrich egg, some animal bones, and a theodolite [whatever that was to this small boy] picked up during a military career abroad). It was true; I spent hours looking in that cabinet and dreaming.

In other words, he somehow understood what this small boy was interested in. He introduced me to Goethe, Wegener, D'Arcy Thompson and Solly Zuckerman.

In 1942, aged 9 and knowing nothing of Goethe's Faust, I totally 'bought' Goethe's idea that the skull was simply a series of fused vertebrae. Goethe wrote to a colleague:

> *"I have found neither gold nor silver,*
> *but something that unspeakably delights me, Eureka!*
> *Only, I beg of you, not a word*
> *for this must be a great secret!*
> *It is the keystone to human evolution."*

That excited me. I did not know that others had also had this idea (e.g., Oken). Nor did I know that it was technically wrong, until I later came to read Gavin de Beer's tome on the vertebrate skull at university in 1954. Goethe and Oken were both wrong, but so nearly right! Today's developmental biology shows that Goethe and Oken were a little bit more right than most thought at the time, though, of course, for the wrong reasons.

In 1942, also, I may have been the only person in the world who knew about the movements of the continents but did not know that Wegener's beginning-of-the-20th-century ideas were not accepted. When I reached university in 1952, the movements of the continents (plate tectonics) were center-stage. I could not understand the excitement. I had always known it was so!

In 1942, I could not possibly understand the mathematical formulae, as well as Greek and Latin quotations (untranslated), in D'Arcy Thompson's (Figure 2.1) wonderful book *On Growth and Form*. But there is so much in that book to touch a nine-year-old.

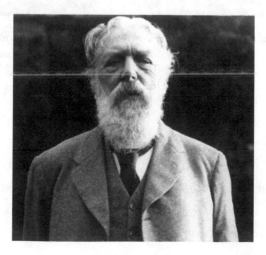

Figure 2.1: D'Arcy Thompson.

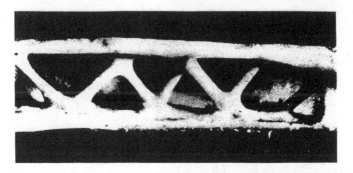

Figure 2.2:   Interior of a vulture's wing bone from D'Arcy Thompson.

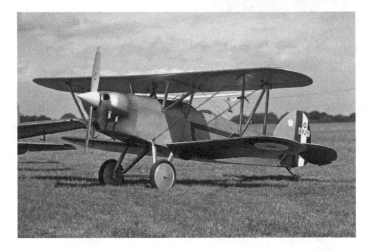

Figure 2.3:   A forerunner to the Spitfire, with struts between the wings just like (as a small boy saw it) the struts within the wings of the bird. Of course, I had it wrong!

For example, the struts in the interior of a bird's wing (Figure 2.2) were so like the struts in the wings of the biplanes during my childhood days (Figures 2.3 and 2.4).

This was all so exciting to a boy whose father worked on the Spitfire, first at Supermarine Works, Southampton, before the war,

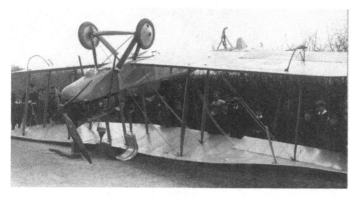

Figure 2.4: It doesn't always work. A forerunner of the Spitfire that landed upside down!

and later, during the war, as Vickers Armstrong's Representative for Scotland on the Ministry of Aircraft Production.

And again, D'Arcy Thompson's pictures showing the similarity between animal backbones and bridges were fascinating. Of course, I was especially aware of the bridge over the river Forth, just down the Firth, from our home in East Lothian (Figure 2.5).

It was, however, Thompson's Cartesian coordinate transformation diagrams used to compare the shapes of faces (from Albrecht Durer, Figure 2.6) and of fishes (D'Arcy Thompson, Figure 2.7) that excited me most. Using this idea, Thompson described differences between animals.

Years later in the 1960s, with pencil and paper (as did Durer and Thompson) I used Cartesian transformations to compare differences in shoulder blades in monkeys and apes. My contribution was double — I borrowed the idea of the transformation to compare bone forms.

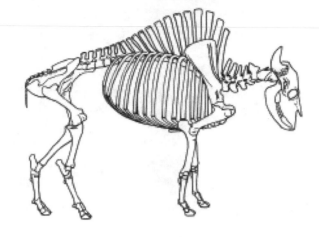

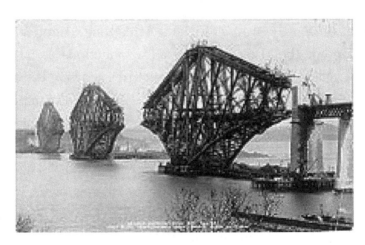

Figure 2.5:   D'Arcy Thompson's comparison of the (above) vertebral column of a bison compared to (below) the cantilever structure of the Forth Bridge under construction.

And I used them to suggest bone functions (Figure 2.8). With Gene Albrecht, originally my student in Chicago in the sixties, I employed them 40 years later (in the form of computational thin plate splines) and (happily) got a similar result

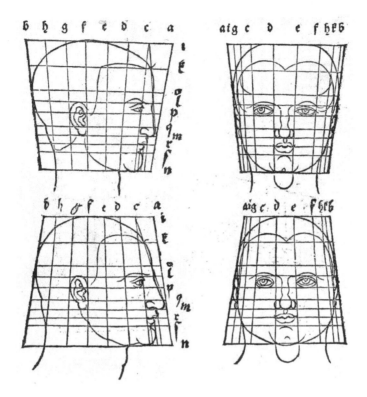

Figure 2.6:   Comparisons of faces (Albrecht Durer as cited by D'Arcy Thompson).

(Figure 2.9). These ideas have been with me ever since reading that book as a schoolboy.

Much more recently, Paul O'Higgins (at the University of York) and I used these ideas to compare skulls of humans and apes (Figures 2.10 and 2.11). Incredible complexities of form are revealed.

I later followed up these studies using many other methods: laser-generated Fourier functions, computer-generated fast

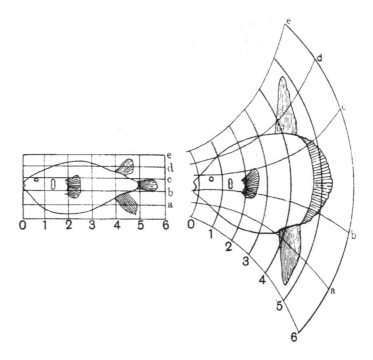

Figure 2.7:   Cartesian transformations of fishes by D'Arcy Thompson, 1917.

Fourier transforms, Buckminster Fuller's 'tensegrity' concepts, engineering finite element analyses, and Thom's catastrophe theory. It was also fascinating how, once again, the science (Figure 2.12) mirrored the art (Figure 2.13)!

Finally, there was that 1934 book by Dr. Zuckerman (as he was then): *The Functional Affinities of Man, Monkeys and Apes*. It completely fascinated me. Thus, in 1933, the then Dr. Zuckerman wrote:

"New students will accept without question evolutionary relationships in which the anatomical differences between two separate types may be less than the differences between two specimens of a single type ... [from which] they may automatically draw distorted evolutionary conclusions."

CARTESIAN TRANSFORMATION: PAPIO INTO GORILLA

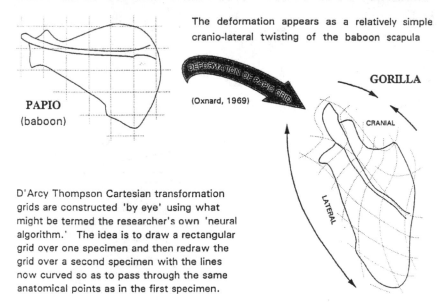

The deformation appears as a relatively simple cranio-lateral twisting of the baboon scapula

PAPIO
(baboon)

(Oxnard, 1969)

GORILLA

CRANIAL

LATERAL

D'Arcy Thompson Cartesian transformation grids are constructed 'by eye' using what might be termed the researcher's own 'neural algorithm.' The idea is to draw a rectangular grid over one specimen and then redraw the grid over a second specimen with the lines now curved so as to pass through the same anatomical points as in the first specimen.

THIN-PLATE SPLINE: PAPIO WARPED ONTO GORILLA

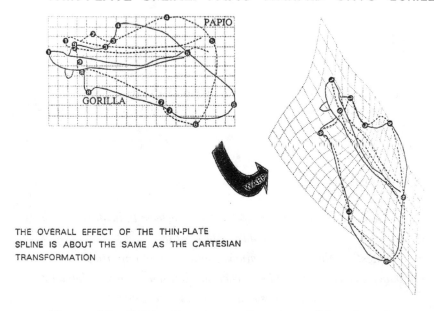

PAPIO

GORILLA

THE OVERALL EFFECT OF THE THIN-PLATE SPLINE IS ABOUT THE SAME AS THE CARTESIAN TRANSFORMATION

Figures 2.8 and 2.9: Cartesian transformations and thin plate splines.

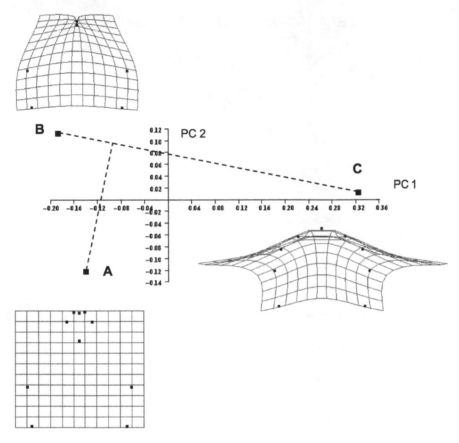

Figure 2.10:   Illustration of the simplicity of differences in skull shape between (A) humans, (B) chimpanzees, and (C) gorillas when based upon geometric landmarks defining simple lengths and widths.

He went on to point out that:

"Anatomical differences are perhaps the least indicators
of evolutionary relationships
... a host of other differentiations could be more important ...
reproductive mechanisms, blood reactions, brain workings, behaviour
patterns, genetics of affinity and divergence,
even diseases and parasites."

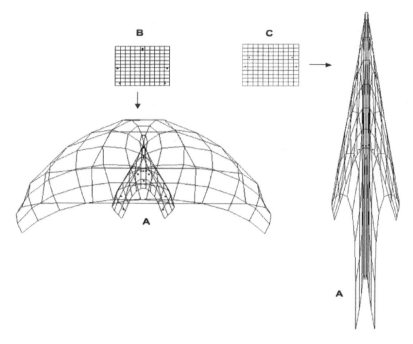

Figure 2.11:   Illustration of the complexities of these same skull shapes when based upon biological landmarks related to bone and muscle attachments reflecting growth and function.

How percipient these words from 1933 sound in the light of today's understanding of evolution. Of course, I then knew little of this; but even then, I was excited by these words!

Neither I, nor that headmaster, knew that I would later work with 'Dr.' Zuckerman!

I thus owe so much to that headmaster! I am sure he had no idea of the stimulus he gave me. I often wonder how little we, as teachers, realize of the impact of our words, sometimes just off-the-cuff remarks, on the lives of our students.

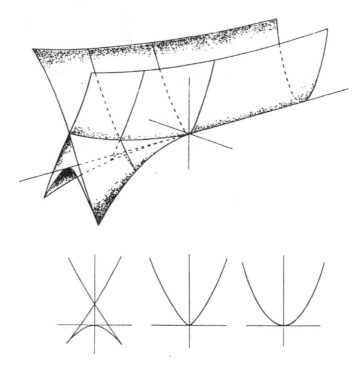

Figure 2.12:   Catastrophe figures.

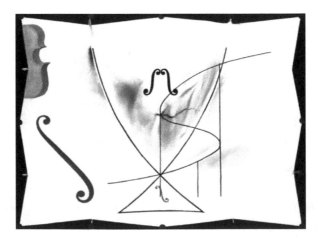

Figure 2.13:   A catastrophe figure in a painting by Salvador Dali.

Secondary School Science Teachers: Biology, Chemistry, Physics

This passion for science was also later stoked in England, where we returned after the war. Thus, as sixth-form schoolboys at Wolsingham Grammar School in Weardale, County Durham, we were told that we had a new teacher for biology, for the last two weeks of term. What can one do in just two weeks, we wondered. The teacher must have wondered too!

That teacher was a woman, very unusual in the sciences in those days! She was, moreover, not long out of college. Indeed, this was possibly her first job. There were only six of us, all boys with raging hormones, in the lower sixth form, as it was called, all hoping to go to university at the end of the following year. All of us wanted to do science of some sort, and two of us wanted to do medicine. We wondered what was going to happen in those last two weeks.

The new teacher, Rosemary Saunders (Rosie, as we immediately called her), came into the room, a small one but with gradually stepped seats like a mini lecture theatre, which was unusual in a school. She plonked a fat book onto the teacher's desk.

"I'm going to read you a story," she said. We looked unbelievingly at each other, and then she started reading. It was *The Worst Journey in the World* by Apsley Cherry-Gerrard.

We were captured and captivated by that 'scientific adventure' book for that entire last fortnight of term. How very, very, clever of her!

She finished that year and taught us for another. She was interested in the field project that I was carrying out at 'Perch Pond' near Frosterley. She even went there to see what I was doing. A report on a personal project was required for the highest marks in biology. (Incidentally, there were no perch in Perch Pond, only a pond at the bottom of a disused limestone quarry, and as the quarry has been re-quarried recently, my Perch Pond is now 'high up in the air'!). Rosie was fantastic. We thought she was the daughter of Professor Saunders, one of the authors of our biology textbook: Borrodaile, Potts and Saunders.

We were taught chemistry by Mr. Brown, who had a face covered with scars (the results of chemical explosions, we found out). He had no hesitation in taking us well beyond the normal chemistry curriculum. We made nitrogen triiodide in a practical class and got enormous pleasure out of placing it on the floor along the corridor so that it would explode when the girls in other classes (there were no girls in chemistry in those days) were walking past! (This is naughty today, and probably was then too.)

Mr. Brown introduced us to parts of chemistry outside the curriculum, such as the organic colour tests. It was just fancy, learning stuff outside the curriculum! This knowledge would have been of no use if I had done the Higher School Leaving Certificate chemistry practical examination in school, because the school lab didn't have the reagents. But for some reason, our examination was held in the university lab, so the special reagents were all on their shelves. As a result, I was able to provide far better answers to the practical questions (identifying the presence of a benzene ring, as I remember it) than was expected!

We were taught physics by Mr. Hewitt. He, too, introduced us to matters that were outside the curriculum. One problem from the final practical examination involved an electric circuit and a pendulum with a plumb bob that was also a magnet oscillating in the earth's field. The curriculum expected us to know these items separately, but not to use them together in a practical test where we did not know the answer. Fascinating!

In all the sciences thus, we were introduced to thinking far beyond the curriculum, and to thinking where we did not know the answer. All six of us went on to university, among whom two went to medical school!

Yet More Teachers: Reading, Writing, Speaking, Acting

But it was not just the sciences that Wolsingham Grammar School gave me. We had a wonderful English teacher, Miss Potts (later Mrs. Bainbridge), who enormously influenced me through reading, writing, speaking and acting.

I had already learnt *the pleasure of reading* from the 'Heid Yin', but Miss Potts certainly reinforced it in spades. She had me read about the life of Florence Nightingale. I had thought Florence Nightingale was 'just a nurse' — a puerile idea! That book let me see what a powerful woman she was, especially how she used numbers, statistics and visual plots to pursue her case.

I hesitate to mention my writing because I am sure I now have many writing habits that Miss Potts would not have liked. I especially remember writing a school essay titled: 'Should Britain become the 50th State of the USA?' I wrote a brilliant (in my opinion) essay taking the 'Yes' position (which is interesting in view of our later translation to America, and now Brexit!), but I was given a 'D' for that essay. The teacher (not Miss Potts) just did not like the position I took. Perhaps this was my first bit of 'heretical' writing; a theme that I have continued most of my life. So, I likewise learnt *the pleasure of writing* from Miss Potts. I have since written many academic books; they don't make much money!

Of course, acting is also important to an academic. This came from my parts in the school plays that Miss Potts directed. One year I was 'Inspector of Schools', a lesser part in Gogol's *The Government Inspector*. The next year I was a major character, Archbishop Beckett, in Eliot's *Murder in the Cathedral*.

I have never forgotten the dress rehearsal. There was one point in the play where the cathedral monks knew the four knights were coming to murder Beckett. They had to go around shouting, "Bar the doors!" But I, as Beckett, wanted to be a martyr, so I had to call for them to unbar the doors.

I had to shout, "Unbar the door," and then again, in a louder voice, "unbar the door," and finally in an exceedingly loud shout, "open the door!" I had difficulty in shouting on stage. Miss Potts had to show me how to do it. At the dress rehearsal a small boy, after the final shout of "OPEN THE DOOR," said one more word: **"RICHARD!"** (Figure 2.14).

The entire cast and the dress rehearsal audience collapsed. Miss Potts threatened anyone with a fate worse than death if they said that on the night! Thus, did I learn *the pleasure of acting*.

Acting, and entertaining one's audience, is so important to a teacher. Entertainment aids teaching and learning so very much. Death to dumb boring lectures we have all sat through! I can still recite large chunks of *Murder in the Cathedral*, *The Rhyme of the Ancient Mariner*, *The Lambton Worm*, *The Blaydon Races*, and of course, Shakespeare: "Let me have men about me that are fat..." and even "By the cruel gods, 'tis most ignobly done to pluck me by the beard..." and so on. Everyone in our family leaves the room when I feel the urge to recite!

Finally, Miss Potts made me Chairman of our School Literary and Debating Society. We had a mock election (at the same time as a national election) and I stood as the Conservative Candidate. *And I won* (in labor, coal-mining, socialist, almost communist County Durham, no less!).

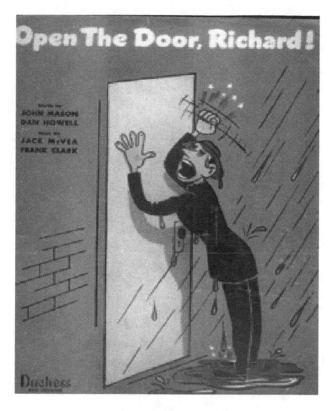

Figure 2.14: "Open the door, Richard, open the door and let me in!" A 1947 pop sensation by Jack McVea and His All Stars.

I displayed a poster with the theme:

*"Our **E**rni**E**, for **E**ducation, **E**mancipation, and **E**quality"*

with emphasis on the very large letter '**E**'s. I was the only candidate who had a poster, but as my fellow students didn't know my middle name was Ernest, it did not achieve the effect I had hoped for.

I especially remember my final speech before the vote. I described a society where one would be looked after from cradle to grave. A socialist idea, as I put it. The audience were puzzled, thinking I was starting to support the opposition (the Labour Party). In concluding, however, I let on to the audience that the society I had described was slavery in the United States; my description of socialism!

The following year I ran as the Communist Candidate. To my amazement, I once again got in! But I never mentioned this while emigrating, years later, to the United States. Thus, did I learn *the pleasure of speaking*, also very important for a budding academic.

Even Teachers Out of School

But it was not just regular school teachers who taught me. There were also Sunday school teachers and the Methodist chapels throughout the north-country dales.

One woman ran a very active Sunday school at Bridgend Methodist Chapel in my home village, Frosterley. She started a fantastic youth club (she even attained local government funds for this!) and supported the Methodist Eisteddfods that were run throughout Weardale. She put on pantomimes at Christmas (I often played the 'Demon King' or 'The Dame'), and was in comedies (farces) at other times of the year.

Further, we had debates, essay writings, recitations, and singing (though I was usually hidden in the middle of the choir; my singing voice was not very good).

And this now amazes me — she encouraged me into local preaching! Although there had been a Union of Methodist Churches much earlier that century, it was not really consummated in Weardale. In Weardale, Wesleyan, Primitive, Baptist and Ebenezer had all remained separate. As the single minister preached in a circuit, there was no one to speak in the other chapels at other times. Thus, lay preachers were used, and I became one!

My 'sermons' (really only 15-minute mini-sermons as I probably could not be trusted with the whole thing) were usually about science and medicine. How I wove these into the chapel services, I can't now imagine. Though I do remember one talk I gave to the 'Women's Bright Hour!', contrasting the seven wonders of the ancient world with those of the modern! I even showed my own sketches of the 'wonders'; no slides, power points or videos in those days!

This was all great fun. *I owe so much to that Sunday school teacher, Miss Jenny Reed, to Bridgend Methodist Chapel, and to the entire village of Frosterley.*

I especially remember a friend named Colin Gowland. We were very evenly matched at badminton, but we were later separated by what I now know was a sudden subarachnoid haemorrhage. *So sad, so especially sad for his new wife and baby-to-come (whom his wife named Corinne!).*

First Surgical Operations (Without a License!)

I even performed my first surgical operation (probably illegally and hopefully covered by the statute of limitations!) in Weardale. One older villager (Willie Walton, sister of Maggie Walton who ran Bridge-End store) knew lots about animals, so the local farmers went to him before spending money on a vet. When Willie knew that I was bound for medical school, he introduced me to some of his 'secrets'. For example, a sheep might be found walking in circles, either right or left. If left untreated, such animals invariably died.

But he had a secret treatment! He had a most beautiful brass Victorian trephine (Figures 2.15 and 2.16). "If you draw lines from the horn to the edge of the eye and the root of the

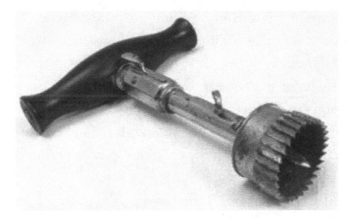

Figure 2.15:   An old trephine, but not the one used by Willie Walton; his was far finer!

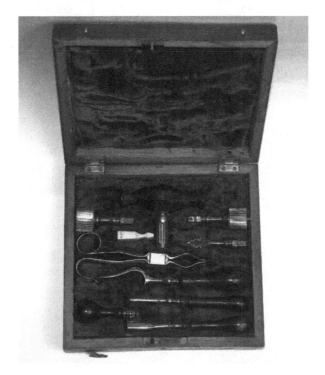

Figure 2.16:   Victorian instruments for brain surgery, including a trephine. Brain surgery then!

ear, you make a mark, and that is where you cut," he said. After removing a bone disc, a feather (!) passed into the skull and whisked around might find a parasite. If there was, then you put the disc of bone back and put a little tar on it. The sheep would get better, or not.

If, however, you did not find a parasite, then you did it again on the other side! I don't know his mortality rate, but if you did nothing they all died. So, it may have been useful.

Willie also had a treatment for 'rheumatism' in 'beasts'. 'Beasts', of course, were cattle. And I never knew what he meant by rheumatism! His treatment was to make a hole through the dewlap at the front of the cow, push a piece of fennel grass through it and tie it in a knot! There would be a violent inflammatory reaction around it (as I now know). Whether the cow got better or not, I don't know.

He told me, again secretly, that you could do the same thing for rheumatism in people! You made the hole in the ear lobe and pushed a piece of fennel grass through it. I don't know if he ever did it; he may have been leg pulling. I was green in those days. Perhaps I still am!

And when I worked on Dobson's farm near 'White Kettle' (real name: White Kirkley) to make money in the summer, I was always given the medical jobs.

I was the one who removed ticks from the fleece of a sheep. I was the one who had to cut the horn off some 'owd tupp' (the horn growing back into its face). I was the one who was shouted at to catch the lamb as it escaped from its handlers. But how does a neophyte catch a runaway lamb? Why, by the horns, of course..? And then the horns came off in my hand, and the horn cores bled furiously. But the lamb didn't seem to notice. Nobody told me!

I was also the one that had to drive the tractor — an old Davy Brown. Of course, I could not drive. But it seems on the farm that did not matter. The first day I drove it around until, after about two hours, it came to a sudden grinding halt. I had no idea what was wrong. I was tempted to open the bonnet, but the presence of steam warned me! It turned out that that old tractor had a manual blind that had to be opened by hand to cool the engine after one had driven it for a little while. Nobody told me.

Applying to Medical School: Decisions, Decisions, Decisions

My father had passed for grammar school at age 11, but then was taken out at 12 to work because of the Great Depression. He was cross about this for his whole life! Hence, he was determined that his children would not miss out on education. My mother, having been a nurse in the days after the First World War, was naturally biased toward medicine. But in the small village where we lived, we did not know how to go about it!

In those days, the decision to do medicine — or indeed any university subject — had to be made very early. If one did not pass the examination at age 11 (the 'eleven-plus') to go to grammar school, one was almost forever denied the chance of a university education.

And, having passed the eleven-plus, if one did not, a year later, enter the 'Latin' stream, one could not go to medical school (it was thought that physicians, like lawyers, should know Latin!). It was only later that I realized how many different 'Latins' there are: Literary Latin (of Vergil), church Latin, legal Latin, medical

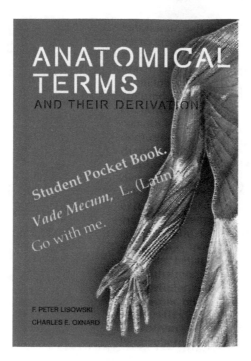

Figure 2.17:   New help for new students. Professor Peter Lisowski and I wrote a little book for medical students. This book is especially useful to students (often foreign) with no classical education.

Latin, even schoolboy Latin of De Bello Gallico Caesaris (*"Caesar ad sum iam forti, Cicero ad erat!"*) (Figure 2.17).

Likewise, in grammar school, if at the age of 14 one chose geography instead of biology, and art instead of chemistry, one was also unlikely to be allowed to do medicine. And what silly choices! Chemistry rather than art I could partly understand, although even then I knew that the creativity of art is so much related to the creativity of science. But geography instead of biology? The two go together: Biogeography, geographical biology, human geography!

Finally, in the sixth form of grammar school (16–18 years), if one wanted medical school, one had to take biology, chemistry and physics, and obtain very high marks to wit. In Scotland, of course, this was relaxed, but at the penalty of doing an extra year of science at university (which was probably not a bad idea!).

In Wolsingham Grammar School (founded in 1614!), medical school-bound students usually went to Kings College, Newcastle (now Newcastle University) upon winning county major university scholarships. But a few Wolsingham students had not gone to Kings College! Geoff Oates, the son of our headmaster (needless to say, we always knew our Headmaster as 'Titus'), had very high marks, obtained a state scholarship, and entered Birmingham University Medical School. Therefore, when I also obtained a state scholarship (which allowed me to go to any university), following Geoff Oates seemed a good way to go. Other students, like John Backhouse before me and Geoff Harrison after me, also got 'states' and went to Birmingham. What a way to choose a medical school!

Having decided on Birmingham, I applied there and I didn't apply anywhere else. I thought that if I wanted to go there, that was where I should apply. I was called for interview.

The Interview, and the Result!

Problem: it was close to Christmas, and I was the Demon King in our local village pantomime. With long thin claw-like fingers, green makeup and a ghoulish cackle, I loved scaring the little kids sitting on the floor at the front of the stage. The show was in the evening, so in order to go for my interview at 9.00 am the next morning, I had to take the night train from Weardale in County Durham to Birmingham in the Midlands.

In those days, unlike the furious night bus in Harry Potter, the night train was very slow. We stopped at every station to load or unload agricultural products, and we spent two hours in Crewe. In the words of the old song:

> *"Oh, Mister Porter, what shall I do,*
> *I wanted to go to Birmingham,*
> *But they've taken me on to Crewe."*

When I arrived in Birmingham, I just had time to wash and brush up in the station toilets before getting to the medical school, hungry and breathless. I was ushered into the interview. Several venerable-looking men were at a long table, and I was 'below the salt'. The entire interview involved only one person (Professor Smout, Sub-Dean of Medicine).

He was quite grumpy. His first question was:

"What does your father do for a living?"

I think he expected my father to be a doctor! He asked three other inconsequential questions, but nothing about my interests in university, science, medicine, or people. Finally, he concluded, even more grumpily: "I see you have only applied to one medical school! Don't you think that was foolish?"

But when I got home, a telegram from Professor Smout was waiting for me (no e-mails in those days).

It was dated the day before my interview!

And it said that I was accepted! I was so cross, but also, of course, enormously relieved! I was determined never to have anything to do with medical student admissions ever again. But I was all set to meet the cast of characters, students, teachers, researchers and practitioners of the next stage of the passion.

3 First Discovery: A Very Small Finding

As is evident from Chapter 2, I had, from a very early age, been interested in the anatomy of the human body. But human anatomy was gradually transforming into a (politically incorrect) 'science of man', later to become 'human biology' and later still 'human science'. I thought all this must surely relate to medicine. I read some of the classics, one of which was Engels (1866). His words on changes in science (modified) describe my idea of changes in anatomy.

> *"Anatomy, up to the end of the 18th century, was predominantly a*
> *collecting science:*
> *a science of finished things.*
> *In my century, the 20th century, it has become, predominantly, a*
> *developing science,*
> *a science of unfinished things.*
> *In your, my reader's, century, in which I am just an old interloper, it*
> *is an interpretative science,*
> *a science of new things,*
> *It now hopes to bind everything, eventually, into one great whole."*

When I actually arrived in 1952 as a medical student in Birmingham, I realized that Sub-Dean Professor Smout, my interviewer in the process of applying to medical school (Chapter 2), was only Acting Head of Anatomy during the war. Professor Solly Zuckerman, though appointed Professor and Head of Anatomy in

1938, was involved in the war effort and only took up the post at war's end.

Of course, Zuckerman was a top-notch scholar, but he almost never appeared in the dissecting room. It was rumored among the students that he knew no anatomy! Early one morning, however, he did come in. I may have been one of a very small number of students actually dissecting so early in the day. He pointed at me: "You, I want you to come and dissect a chimpanzee."
(Of course, not the whole chimpanzee but one part of it, relevant to some research in which he was engaged at that time.)

So, I did. As a result, I actually made a small discovery.

A Missing Muscle?

After dissecting the chimpanzee's chewing muscles in which Zuckerman was interested, I discovered that the jaw muscle was fleshy (dark in the diagram, Figure 3.1), whereas the human jaw muscle had a silvery tendon (white in the diagram).

How could these be so different; weren't chimpanzees and humans closely related?

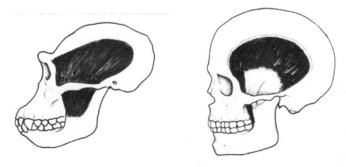

Figure 3.1:   The outside of one jaw-closing muscle in a chimpanzee and a human.

Then I had two ideas. Perhaps, in chimpanzees, the tendon of the human *was not missing*, but rather *it was just hidden deep inside*. Or perhaps in humans, the outer fleshy muscle, so evident in the chimpanzee, *was truly missing!*

I made a cut down through the muscle in the chimpanzee. This revealed that the tendon was indeed present. It was just buried underneath a large entirely fleshy superficial muscle (left frame of Figure 3.2) that the human seemed not to have!

The tendon in the chimpanzee was not missing!
The chimpanzee's outer fleshy muscle was missing in humans!

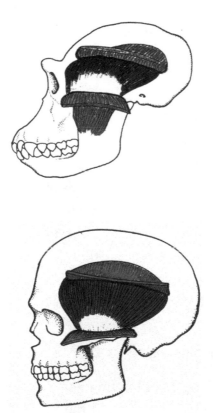

Figure 3.2:   Deep to the superficial muscle in a chimpanzee was indeed a muscle with a silvery tendon (like humans). And in the occasional human, right, I found thin outside muscle covering the muscle with the tendon (like chimpanzees).

Almost immediately a lucky find in the dissecting room showed that the outer fleshy muscle of the chimpanzee was indeed (occasionally) present (though very thin) in humans (Figure 3.2 right frame).

The muscle in humans may not be missing!
Chimpanzees did not have a tendon missing; it was humans that had
a muscle missing!

It is such a small finding, but incredibly exciting to a beginning student. Finding something no one else knew! I think, in that fraction of a second, I was really hooked on research.

It seemed that, on occasion, the chimpanzee condition could appear as an anomaly in humans: *a ghost, perhaps, of an earlier stage in evolution, or a mistake in an earlier stage of development, or both!*

But why? At the time, I thought that this reduction in the chewing muscle in humans might be related to the reduced chewing of relatively soft foods in humans, as compared with the long hard chewing of the tough fibrous foods of chimpanzees.

However, whatever I thought might be the cause at the time, this discovery led on to the further discovery that although humans differed from chimpanzees in lacking this particular muscle, the other non-muscular, collagenous, fascial sheets, aponeuroses, and intramuscular tendons were still present.

More Missing Muscles

This led me thinking about the function, development and evolution of both the muscle tissue and the non-muscular connective tissue parts: fasciae, ligaments, tendons and bones.

For example, like human jaw muscles, the human upper limb muscles (Figure 3.3), again alone among other primates, are not involved in the big mechanical forces of locomotion as in apes and monkeys.

Just as I guessed that human jaw muscles needed to be less powerful because of the softer human diets compared with apes and monkeys, so perhaps, I thought, human upper limb muscles needed to be less powerful because upper limbs are not involved powerfully in locomotion (as they are in apes and monkeys). Perhaps, in humans, parts of these muscles were lost. Yet variations in humans exist on occasion: again, possibly, *ghosts of times past, from development, or evolution?*

I then surmised that this idea could be tested by looking at the lower limbs. The lower limbs, though working differently in humans as compared with apes and monkeys, still participate in

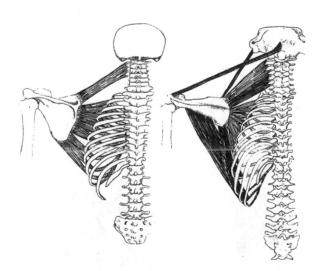

Figure 3.3:   One muscle sheet holding the shoulder blade in humans (left frame) compared with the same muscle sheet in an ape (right frame). The 'extra' muscles, darker in the ape, all exist as rare variations in humans. The diagrams are 'exploded' so that all muscles can be seen.

powerful locomotion movements (even if differently: on two limbs as compared with four).

Figure 3.4 shows that, indeed, there are differences in the lower limb muscles between apes and humans, but not *missing differences* like those evident in the upper limbs and jaws. In other words, a mark of walking on our lower limbs only (in contrast to apes and monkeys) may be as evident in weaker arms with lost muscles, as in stronger legs without muscle loss!

Years later I came to understand that the genes and molecules responsible for generating muscle tissues are different from those responsible for forming connective tissues. Interference with muscle-generating molecules may eliminate muscle tissue. Yet connective tissues within and around muscles are still present as connective-tissue molecules are still functioning!

Of course, these explanations are due to turn-of-the-century findings. However, the implications were evident to

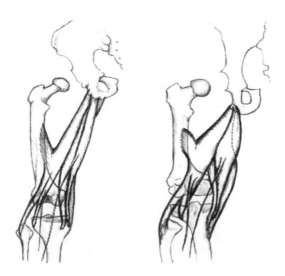

Figure 3.4:   Although the muscles are different in humans (left) and apes (gorillas, right), there are no special missing muscles in the human hip and thigh. Again, the diagrams are 'exploded'.

me even in the 1950s. But then, developmental biology was just its progenitor, embryology; cell biology had only just been recognized and was a small part of histology; molecular biology had scarcely been invented. And the full DNA story was for the far future.

To me, as a beginning researcher, it was so exciting to see far ahead from that very first discovery. However small, it was my very first assay into real research.

But Still 'Only' a Medical Student

However, at the time of the jaw muscle finding, I was still only a little medical student. My question became: how could a medical student do research? The answer came from Zuckerman.

Each year, a few medical students would be selected to study for an honors bachelor's degree in science. Such an intercalated undergraduate degree was not unknown — there were several medical schools where one could take such advanced courses in the basic medical sciences.

Zuckerman's unique idea, however, was that that year should be only research. No didactic courses! No lectures (except research lectures by visitors)! No learning the recipes of techniques! No cramming! No written examinations! His students, even though just 19-year-old undergraduates, were to be thrown into real research. If we needed a technique, we learnt it or invented it; but not otherwise. And at the end we had to write a thesis and take an oral examination from experts in the area.

My thesis included the structure and development of the face. Professor Alan Boyd (of Hamilton, Boyd and Mossman fame) was the world's expert in this area. I was terrified to discover that he was one of my external examiners.

Today, such research courses are regularly available in the best medical schools, but in Birmingham at that time it was new. One had to apply to enter the course, and one had to take a separate examination to test one's aptitude for research. If successful, one received a whole year's scholarship superadded to one's five-year state scholarship.

So popular — and so prestigious — in those days was the idea of getting this extra honors degree that more than half the medical class opted for the examination. Can we really see fifty percent of today's medical students taking an additional examination(!), success in which would delay qualifying in medicine by a further year(!), thereby reducing their lifetimes' emoluments by those of the most highly paid last year(!)?

That examination was especially interesting: seven essay questions, but we only had to answer one. And we had three whole hours for that one. Never had I had so much choice, nor so much time!

Six of the questions were like those in the regular anatomy examinations, only more complex, involving matters outside the usual curriculum, and especially ideas that were not well worked out. Imagine the *angst* among students today if questioned outside the curriculum!

There was no cry of:
"Will it be on the test?"
from the students of that time!

One question, however, was different from the others. It ran thus:
"In the days of Malpighi, science was supported by private patrons. Today it is state-aided. Discuss." Was it an accident that the six of

us who won that year all answered that particular question? Was it an accident that one of Zuckerman's interests was the funding of science? *Was it an accident that such a question could not possibly have been 'spotted'?* I learnt so much in that research year, even though the research I carried out was just old-fashioned classical anatomy. After all, it was only 1954.

Therefore Next: BSc in Science (Not Medicine)!

For my honors BSc, I thought of examining the anatomy of the twelve cranial nerves. A moment's thought said it was too big a task. So, I decided to examine only one cranial nerve: the fifth. A few days' reading showed that even that was too big a project. Finally, I decided to look at only one branch of that nerve: the maxillary, leading to the infraorbital nerve, passing through the orbit and onto the face — this after a fortnight's reading. So were our student enthusiasms cut down (Figure 3.5).

Obviously, I could examine human material from our dissecting room. And I had access to apes and monkeys from the collections in the Birmingham department and from the Natural History Museum, South Kensington.

But I thought the problem was wider than just primates. How different were these nerves in animals with amazing sensory abilities in the face, the very extensive sensory organ of the trunk tip in elephants, in the melon in whales, to the nerves to the huge vibrissae of the seal (Figure 3.6)?

But there were also other possibilities. I decided to examine common or garden mammals like horses. Where could I get horses?

It turned out that Dr. (later Professor) Eric Ashton knew. He had worked on the olfactory abilities of dogs (to sniff out mines)

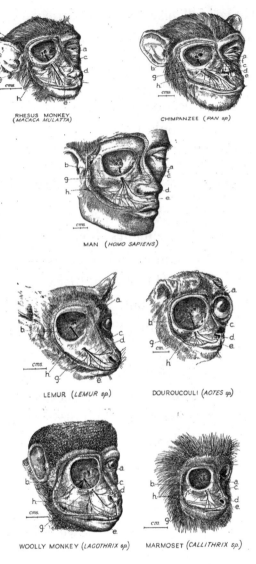

Figure 3.5:   Nerves in the faces of a human, an ape, and various other primates.

at Melton Mowbray (classified military work). He knew, too, that Melton Mowbray was the home of the cavalry. Horses die; we could have heads! (That worried me: all I knew of Melton Mowbray were the pies. Where did the meat come from, I wondered?)

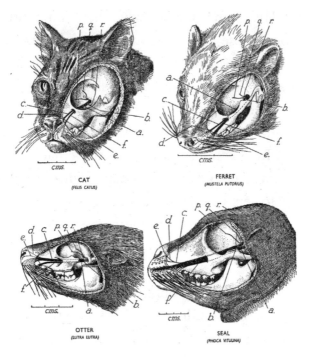

Figure 3.6:   Nerves in the faces of some mammals.

Ashton would take me to pick up some horse heads. Ashton's car was a Hillman Minx and he proposed putting several horse heads in the boot. I remonstrated with him.

"Horses' heads are very big; you'll only get one in the boot,"
I said.
"Rubbish,"
he said.
"You can get a whole man in there."
To demonstrate, he jumped in and closed the lid. Of course, the lid was self-locking and he had the key in his pocket.
"Get the other key from my white coat in my room in anatomy,"
came the muffled cry from the boot.

So, I did. His room was just above the main entrance to the medical school. I chose a pathway to his room by entering a back door of the school, traversing every corridor and every floor, accidentally(?) alerting everyone as to the situation, and eventually ending up at his room. I returned to the car brandishing the key, to find every member of the department down by the car encouraging Ashton that I was coming. The sort of story that lives in legend!

Of course, dissecting very large animals involves problems in preservation. However much formalin I used, those heads, in a huge tank in my room, stank. Of course, it was not MY room; it was for all six honors students. But it became *my* room; the stink was so great.

To reduce the smell, I would work only late at night. Came the night when I was standing on a dissecting stool, wielding a rather large manual cutter (no electrical equipment in those days) *attacking* the head of a cow. I was in the dark, with a lamp shining on the specimen. It also lit my face from underneath. The door opened; it was the security man checking. There was a scream. He fled the department, ran from the building, and was never seen again!

I was horrified one day when Zuckerman came around to see my dissections. Hidden behind his back was a huge magnifying glass. Hrrmmmpppphhhhhh, he said, peering through it at my dissections. One of them was one of the horses — not the whole horse of course, just its head, but even that is very large; a magnifying glass was scarcely needed. An interesting ploy, I noted (I have subsequently used it myself on my own students)!

Shortly after this, a small box — very small — appeared upon my desk with a note:

"Please dissect the head of this rare African Shrew, particularly the nerves of the vibrissae."

It was signed: 'SZ'.

I had never dissected anything so small. But I thought about it, borrowed a dissecting microscope and some eye-surgery instruments, and spent two whole days doing that dissection. I was so engrossed that I never noticed that virtually every member of the department dropped in over those two days to see how I was getting on.

That rare African shrew was, of course, a common shrew that had been brought in by a fellow student's cat! Was this Ashton getting his own back? Or one of my fellow students? Surely not Zuckerman?

But something good came out of this prank. I found that I could indeed tease out nerve fibers. And I used this in a later project where I teased individual nerve fibers from monkey cadavers. The result of this research year was a thesis that gave rise, eventually, to four published papers and a number of abstracts and communications to scientific societies. And it continued my link with science when I returned to the standard medical course (see next chapter).

Research after Medicine: Back to Science

It was therefore natural that, after qualifying in medicine and doing the necessary year of hospital house jobs, I would return to work with Sir Solly (as he had become).

He encouraged me to apply for the Biet Memorial Predoctoral Fellowship to help me fund a PhD. I did not know at the time that Solly, himself, had been a former holder. Nevertheless, I did not get it.

However, he did get me a university fellowship. This was actually better for me! It was certainly much more money, for though I was working predoctorally for a PhD degree, that fellowship (following my medical degree) was postdoctoral in level (and salary!). Zuckerman followed this up by appointing me to a tenured lectureship, and then, only three years after that, promoting me to Senior Lecturer. This was an enormously accelerated *cursus honorum* for those days (or, for that matter, for any days). But Zuckerman could work miracles.

Those post-medical degree years with Solly in anatomy were a most seminal period for me.

First, as indicated, I was enabled to get a PhD on top of my BSc and MB, ChB degrees. My eventual thesis was followed by a 100-page monograph and nine published papers, four from when I was an undergraduate — a great start to a research career!

Second, Eric Ashton and I obtained a five-year, one-million-dollar research grant (a lot of money in the sixties) from the US Public Health Service (USPHS). Today, one can only obtain a grant like that if one is collaborating with someone in the US. And that grant was even more valuable than it appears because the USPHS paid infrastructure monies (which in the USA go to the university). But British universities had no mechanism to accept infrastructure money, so that also came to us to spend as research funds. (Let it be clear that we got this grant through Zuckerman's long-standing pre-war, war-time, and post-war connections, see last part.)

One of the usages of this money was the appointment of Dr. Stanley Salmons (now Emeritus Professor in Liverpool University and, in retirement, an author of much fascinating science fiction). He had qualifications in physics and electronic engineering. We wanted him to build miniaturized equipment to obtain radio-telemetric signals of muscle activity and bone strains from living, moving monkeys.

Of course, it became clear that it was a foolish idea at that point. Stanley realized very quickly that miniaturization had not, at that stage, proceeded far enough. It did become possible years later.

But he put his part of the grant to good use, inventing, among other things, the 'buckle transducer' for recording strain in tendons *in vivo*. He collaborated with Dr. Gertha Vrbova (physiology at Birmingham). Much later, as professor at the University of Liverpool, he used non-cardiac muscle (latissimus dorsi) to help bolster heart function in disease.

Serendipity: Amazing Research Materials

During this time, I became involved, completely by accident, in obtaining an absolutely remarkable set of primate materials that became the mainstay of much of the primate part of my lifetime's work. It happened like this.

As I was driving to work one day, I heard on the car radio that there was a fire at Tyseley Pet Stores. It was on my way, so I stopped to see what had happened. As far as I knew, this was a little shop that sold puppies, kittens, guinea pigs and goldfish to small children, or rather, to small children's parents. What I did not know was that, in addition, they imported and sold a wide variety of 'exotic' animals. Totally forbidden today, but it was allowed then!

The fire had suffocated (not burnt) literally thousands of creatures housed in large sheds at the back. There was a tamandua and a flying fox among a number of rare mammals. There were very large numbers of small tropical birds. And there were about a thousand individual primates! These included little samples of the same forms from known localities. Thus, there were about thirty tamarins, ten spider monkeys, eight colobus monkeys, and so on — a handful of specimens of each of about forty different species. This would permit study of variation within species, ranging widely over the primate order, something not possible before.

"What will happen to these carcasses?"
I asked the owner.
"Oh, we'll have to burn them,"
he said.
"I'll give you £100 for the lot,"
I said, and the deal was done.

Two hours later, news of the fire was on the national air waves. The well-known primatologist, John Napier, called from London; *but he was too late*!

Years later, in Australia, I gave a talk about variations in soft tissues in nonhuman primates. An animal rights person was present and she saw my list of materials.
"To get those materials, how many monkeys did you shoot?"
she wanted to know, peremptorily.
I told the above story!

Totally unexpectedly, this had a sad ending. Long after the days of Solly Zuckerman and later John Eayrs as Birmingham Anatomy Department Heads, a molecular biologist became head. Partly because he wanted to mould the department into his own molecular image (fair enough in the mores of those days), but partly because he wanted to eliminate any memory of Solly (he even had a bronze bust of Solly consigned to the dustbin), he ordered those primate carcasses destroyed!

True, they were not molecular data. But did he not realize what a loss this was, even to molecular biology, never mind anatomy?

Molecular biologists today *know* they *need* to know: which dogfish, which lizard, which rabbit, *which monkey*? And for such purposes they need tissues, cells, and even molecules from carcasses!

My doctoral thesis was titled 'Structure and Function in Primates'. As a result of all the data I got from this huge collection of cadavers, I was able to follow it up with many published papers. These were essays into functional anatomy and were, thus, tackling problems probably not very different from many another study of functional anatomy in those days. They were attempting to find out, from the study of the anatomy of living primates, how to estimate ('guesstimate') function in fossil primates.

The new aspects of the work were that large samples, defined by many new measurements, could be studied by (then) new computational methods.

But because studies of fossils were then (and still are) extremely contentious, to avoid the new methods being damned for what they said about fossils, I worked first on the shoulder. Shoulder bones are fragile and rarely fossilized. Thus did I avoid '*goring* someone else's fossil *ox*'!

'World Expert' on the 'Right' Shoulder!

Though I did not fully understand it at the time, this shoulder study (which looked only at the 'right shoulder' to reduce the number of dissections!) would form the basis of a whole radiation of investigations over many years. I started that work with attempts to understand (a) how animals moved and how their shoulders worked during those movements, (b) how those movements were related to the size and disposition of the shoulder muscles, and (c) how the shoulder muscles were associated with the shapes of the shoulder bones and joints.

The steps from animal movements through their muscles to their bones and joints was thus studied explicitly in these many extant species through finding facts.

But the reverse steps, from the forms of partial bones and joints in fossils to possible implications for muscles in fossils, suggest only possible ideas about movements in fossils. They are estimates, not facts. Again:

Facts are chiels that winna ding an' downa be disputed
Rabbie Burns 1759–1796
But facts also can be (and very often are) misused in the 'divinations' of evolution.

"How could one haruspex look another in the face without laughing?"
(Cato 234-149 BC: A haruspex divined the future from anatomy)

As a result, the start of this work involved searching the natural history literature for information about how the monkeys and apes of today move. This was before the days of modern field studies of primates. Such information then was mostly observational and quite non-quantitative.

The same thing applied to the anatomy of the engines of movement, the muscles. Many muscle dissections had been done over many centuries. But again, there were few numbers!

Such studies go back a long way, even to Galen of Pergamum. He provided pictures of the equipment for holding animals for dissection. But he also wrote that:

"It is preferable to use other animals for dissection: the spectacle of the monkey is too hideous"! From which I believe that some 'dissection' of those days was vivisection (Figure 3.7)!

By thinking, Aristotle believed that the brain produced phlegm to cool the heart. But *by doing*, Galen showed that the brain was connected to and controlled the entire body. He wrote:

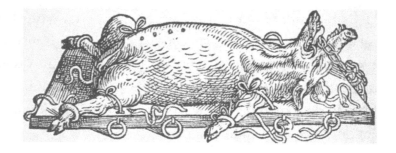

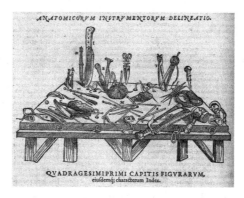

Figure 3.7:   Above, pig prepared for vivisection, and below, dissecting instruments.

"If you press so much upon a cerebral ventricle that you wound it, immediately the living being will be without movement and sensation, without spirit and voice" (vivisection again!).

Most information about muscles in nonhuman primates was likewise descriptive and non-quantitative, and was well catalogued in Ruch's famous Bibliographia Primatologica.

But information about bones was different. Bones had, indeed, been measured many times. But the measures were simple, usually only lengths and breadths, and mostly only the mean of one measure or the ratio of two. Muscles were scarcely measured at all. In other words, extensive though these studies had been over the centuries, putting together such information about the muscles and the bones as they functioned held few numbers. Study was primarily by inference. There was no testing of ideas.

This is not a criticism of the earlier work. Many excellent workers had contributed to this vast array of studies. It is just that mechanisms and philosophies had not developed so far. It was just my great good fortune to start at a time when it was beginning to be possible to do something more about such data even though I could not do them all myself.

How Monkeys Move

Assessing how monkeys move, however, was not within my expertise; I was not trained in animal behavior. I would have been of no use in the field; mosquitoes, leeches, extremes of temperature, high humidity, tropical rainstorms, living under canvas, malaria and dengue fever (this last did fall to a colleague) were not my cup of tea!

But I could analyze the literature. Earlier ways of studying animal function involved, first, describing animal behavior (usually locomotion) as a small number of discrete functional groups (e.g., runners, leapers, bipeds). Second, these functional groups could be related to differences in bone measurements. And third, therefore, the bone measurement in fossils could, in reverse, imply possible fossil function.

This seems, on the face of it, reasonably logical. However, I wanted to go further. One element of this was how we looked at function. It seemed to me unlikely that these overall functional groups (e.g., runner, leaper, biped) would be the important functional descriptors for individual bones and joints. I thought the form of particular bones and joints would be more related to function in their own local anatomical region. Thus, *shoulders* would be better examined in the light of *shoulder function within locomotion* but *hips* in the light of *hip function within locomotion*, and so on.

I also thought that using the functional groups as a basis for comparison was too crude. It seemed to me more likely that the functional groups were merely artificial separations of what were really continuous functional spectra. Would it not be better to examine the species separately, without forcing them into groups? Let groups, if there were any, emerge. The huge collection of primate specimens from Tyseley Pet Stores allowed this, though it was a lot of dissection!

These thoughts turned out to be correct. Functions in shoulders and arms in primates are better described as a band-like spectrum, not separate groups; functions in hips and thighs as a star-shaped continuum, again, not separate groups (see later chapter). Later I even realized that other possibilities existed; I discovered doughnut-shaped arrangements, and even some in more than three-dimensions (Figure 3.8).

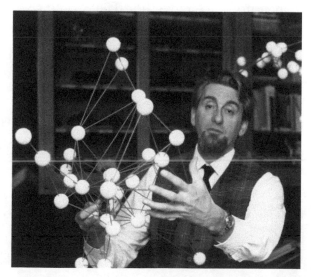

Figure 3.8:   A model requiring more than three dimensions for full representation. Of course, the model itself IS in only three dimensions, but one can see that more than three dimensions are involved because some of the 'distances' (the rods) connecting the species (the 'balls') that should be straight, have to be curved to fit them into just three dimensions! (Compared with an earlier figure, the picture also shows that we gradually age; American students loved my tartan 'weskit'.)

How Bones Work

From muscles to bones: every bone can be described by measurements. An earlier generation of physical anthropologists chose measurements that could be easily taken, such as overall length, overall width, and so on. And these are, indeed, useful measures.

However, given the information about muscles and movements, it seemed that measurements attempting to estimate the mechanical parameters of bones might answer functional questions better. These were measures approximating to muscle leverages, positions of joint axes, bone angles and twists, direction of gravity, and similar mechanically relevant data.

Further, instead of looking at such measures one by one, or perhaps in pairs using simple statistics like means and ratios (all that had already been previously used), it seemed better to try examining all measures taken together. That would give, I thought, a better description of shape, which it did. However, though this did lead to better shape description, and this was the original aim, it led unexpectedly to better functional assessments.

Of course, these all-together-statistics are all very well, but the older non-mathematically inclined biologist doesn't easily grasp them (although today's computer-savvy generations do). So perhaps a first exciting thing was borrowing (from D'Arcy Thompson, Huber, Descartes and others, as described in Chapter 2) an artistic technique for visualizing form: the Cartesian coordinate analysis of D'Arcy Thompson.

For example, using pencil and paper, D'Arcy Thompson showed how the form of one bone could be seen as a simple deformation of another, although there is evidence that his drawings were a little cavalierly!

I, too, used pencil and paper, and was probably also a little cavalierly in my diagrams. But while Thompson was looking at shape deformations that he could see by eye, I was looking at shape differences as they were 'seen' by new statistical axes (also see Chapter 2).

Immediately it seemed I had hit a jackpot. (As an aside, 30 years later, the invention of a computer method known as thin plate splines gave an almost identical result to the original paper and pencil studies; see Chapter 2!)

Thus, studying the shoulder seemed to give a result that, when applied to fossils, revealed functional information.

All nonhuman mammals showed forms of the shoulder that could be described in a continuous spectrum of variation. Humans, and humans alone, lay uniquely separately (Figure 3.9).

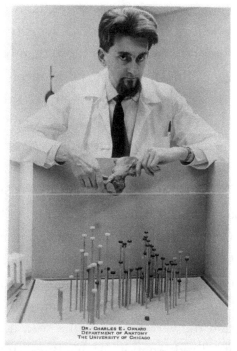

Figure 3.9: A model of the analysis of the shoulder in many mammals. The single small dot at the bottom of the picture is the unique location of humans (with unique shoulder functions). That I am holding a pelvis can be laid at the door of the photographer; he wanted a larger bone!

Presumably, then, any fossil shoulder (if ever one were found) that might be thought to be 'on the way to human functions' might lie appropriately toward the unique position of humans in the model!

I now felt it was necessary to move on from suggesting bone function (as in the above studies) to testing hypotheses about bone function. At first my methods were very simple: armchair guesses of how bones might bear stresses and be strained (more pencil and paper stuff!). This quickly took me, however, into two-dimensional analogs of mechanical function using photoelasticity (borrowed from the Brewsters, father and son, at the beginning of the 19th century).

And then I borrowed real two-dimensional stress and strain analyses from taking engineering courses at the Advanced College of Technology at Salford (now Salford University) in 1962. Even these methods were too crude to give more than ball park ideas in the biological milieu. Bones are just not as nicely geometrical as metal parts! But they did clearly imply that I could, in fact, expect eventually to get better answers. This has now been done.

And by the beginning of the 21st century, even better answers stemmed from three-dimensional stress and strain studies (the 'new biomechanics'). These can now can be combined with the multidimensional statistics (the 'new morphometrics') of today (thanks to Paul O'Higgins at York University and many engineering colleagues at the University of Hull).

The work on the shoulder later expanded to include other bones: hip and thigh, arm and forearm. Later still it included the ankle and foot, and the vertebral column, with a variety of postgraduate students: Fred Anapol, Alana Buck, Jens Hirschberg, A.-T. Hsu, Rob Kidd, and Christine Runnion. I did not study the wrist and hand until several years later (with Russell Tuttle, now

Emeritus Professor at the University of Chicago), perhaps because they are more complicated. And I never even looked at the skull (an even more complex region) until very many years later through work with Pan Ruliang, then from Kunming (the City of Eternal Spring), but now a close colleague in Australia.

The key points in this story, however, are not the actual work that we did, nor especially the particular results that we obtained.

The key points are:

the thinking that we employed,
the tortuosity of the pathway that we took,
the importance of accidental findings along the way, and (very importantly)
the new methods, hypotheses, technologies, and ideas from a range of disciplines, and
the new colleagues inhabiting those disciplines: *physics, mathematics, engineering, geology, and social sciences*, and finally
the wide range of postgraduate students who were attracted to and who elaborated on the ideas.

These links resulted in new research. They made it so exciting. They are among the reasons why I never returned to medical practice.

Time to Move On!

However, having been both student and staff at the same university, the time came when I felt it important to move somewhere else. But where? I therefore had two rather difficult years as I pondered on what I should do next.

I continued to think about where else I could do broader anatomical research. I looked at other UK departments, but they were
mostly *human* anatomy departments. Alec Cave (who had been
one of my doctoral examiners) said he had a readership available
at 'Barts' (St Bartholomew's Hospital Medical School), and that if
I applied I would get it (professors had those kinds of powers in
those days!). But he also advised me not to apply; I think he knew
what was going to happen to anatomy in some of the London medical schools.

So, I looked at departments in the 'British Empire': Canada,
South Africa and Australia. I was just too young for a Chair in
Zoology in Sydney! Nowhere seemed an improvement on
Birmingham. It never crossed my mind to think of the 'Old British
Empire'; that is, the USA!

I therefore matriculated for an external law degree at the
University of London. It was not that I wanted a change of career;
I just thought it was an interesting thing to do. Perhaps it was a dis-
placement activity, and I enjoyed the first year of law very much.
That first year, in those days, comprised of tort, contract, British
constitutional history, and Roman law. Roman law was a whole one
half of the first year! I loved it — it was comparative law, just like
comparative anatomy! *If you want to know about the manumission
of slaves in ancient Rome then I am your man!*

At this point I was invited to give a paper at a symposium at
the University of California, Davis. There I met one of the best
comparative anatomists of those days, Milton Hildebrand. I gave
a highly successful (as I remember it!) paper on my then current
research. At the age of 33 it was my first trip abroad! As a result,
I suddenly realized that there were more than a hundred medical
schools in the US, and that some of them were of very high caliber.

While I was in Davis, the University of Chicago had their spies out (another participant at the Davis conference was Russ Tuttle from Chicago). Almost immediately I had an invitation to visit Chicago for a couple of weeks, together with my wife, Eleanor, to consider taking an appointment there. We went in January, in the depth of winter, but were so taken with what we saw — the staff, the students, the institution, the city — that nine months later, in October 1966, we arrived.

A whole new life awaited!

Most of my Birmingham colleagues could not understand why we went to the USA. Their ideas of Chicago were mainly about the Great Chicago Fire, Al Capone, ghetto riots, freeway traffic jams, and rotting alewives on the lakeshore. They had no idea about the high quality of the University of Chicago, nor about the changes in anatomy being made by Ron Singer, the relatively new Head there.

That anatomy department had long been amongst the best in the US in earlier years, with a number of very well-known faculty. But changes had occurred over the years and the department had gone somewhat downhill as the earlier greats left and/or retired. Singer was providing a new thrust that was moving the department up again. He imported new young faculty and encouraged new research students. He expanded into the research areas that were coming to underlie anatomy. He was moving in the directions that I had already inherited from Zuckerman in Birmingham. Eleanor and I had twelve wonderful years there.

But I had to give up Law — an English Law Degree would not be much use in the USA

4 Chapter First Teaching: The Teaching/Research Nexus

The decision for a career in research inevitably also means a parallel decision for teaching. When that research is medical anatomy, then the teaching includes medical students.

This was one of the reasons why, after qualifying in medicine, I spent two years doing general medicine and surgery, clinical rotations (ear, nose and throat, eyes, skin, obstetrics and gynaecology), and even some locums in general practice. I thought that if I were going to teach medical students, then I ought to have a 'lick' of medical practice, to have some idea how a practicing physician might use anatomy, even if I would not be a practicing physician myself. This has paid off in spades; few anatomy teachers today are medically qualified.

But there is much more to my teaching story than this.

What is Anatomy Good For?

Teaching anatomy, it seems, is quite simple. Listen in lectures, cut in labs, write and talk in exams, get grades, pass. Very clear!

However, it is not just any old anatomy; it's *human* anatomy. We cannot forget the most important component: *humans*. As humans, we walk this earth trying to make something of ourselves and help others along the way (though some denigrate this humanitarian aspect!). Should we not always try to keep our 'humanness': have compassion and benevolence; be well-meaning and kind; and aim to serve rather than just make a profit?

The donors whose bodies are in our anatomy laboratories especially exert their 'humanness', even after death. They are our true mentors and heroes. They help us show humanity in helping others. They make it possible for us and our students to understand the body.

Being able to dissect the human body was both a privilege and a maturation process. We learned how to study the complexity of human structure while building a deep respect for, and connection with, humans. The gift the donors gave us, a gift above anatomical knowledge, was the meaning of being human! What it means to improve life, even from death. How never to forget the human component! The donors led us by example.

Yet for many years now, dissecting the body has been disappearing from the medical curriculum.

This is partly for very good reasons. The entire medical curriculum has become more and more filled with so many new subjects since my day. There is little time for anatomy!

Other good reasons result from technical and pedagogical change. Advances in the technology of anatomy, especially plastination, 3D imaging and printing, and computer teaching, all have provided new learning possibilities, especially those for self-learning.

Anatomy is also disappearing because so much of the old anatomy was based on memorization. Memorization alone often damages the processes of thinking.

A yet further reason for its disappearance is because the medical curriculum is mainly in the hands of educational specialists. They are well experienced at teaching theory, curriculum development, student learning and assessment, and the measurement of outcomes! But they often have no real understanding of anatomy and its value to medical practice.

A final reason is because, in its original usage, the provision of cadavers, of body preparation laboratories, of dissecting rooms, and of, necessarily, only a few students to each teacher around the body and therefore many teachers, is very expensive. Deans of medical schools, struggling under financial woes, have found it easy to save money by eliminating dissection and dissecting laboratories, reducing the body preparation rooms and their attendant preparation staff, getting rid of the staff needed for dissecting-type teaching, and using part-time teaching-only tutors who are so much cheaper (and usefully impermanent!).

However, a different reason for the disappearance of anatomy is a misunderstanding of anatomy's purpose. Just what is anatomy good for?

Surely Anatomy is for Surgery?

One assumption, for example, is that anatomy is for surgery. Anatomy, it is therefore assumed, is not needed by most doctors who will be non-surgical practitioners.

Certainly, anatomy **is critical for surgeons**; even more so in these days of surgical super-specialization. Surgeons now become extremely good, with therefore much reduced morbidity and mortality, by becoming very expert at a small number of (often very complex) procedures. And because surgeons can now 'see' living anatomy in ways not possible before the new imaging tools were developed, knowledge of anatomy is more critical, not less.

However, there is also another 'surgery' — **a 'minor surgery'** — that we sometimes forget: the surgery **of general practice, of emergency medicine, and of the non-specialist**, especially in the country.

This often requires anatomical knowledge in situations where it cannot be quickly looked up. Thus, the 'knife' removing a sebaceous cyst in the neck easily leads to paralysis of a shoulder muscle (trapezius) if knowledge of its nerve supply (the accessory nerve lies very superficially) has been forgotten, (or was never learnt!). The 'needle' in the elbow or buttock readily causes nerve or blood vessel damage if the simple anatomy is absent (or has disappeared!). Even the 'finger' (touching, palpating), the 'eye' (looking, observing), or the 'ear' (hearing, listening) can mislead if what is under the skin has been forgotten (or was never known!).

There was a time when anatomy was so reduced at Harvard Medical School that, in turn, anatomists, pathologists, and eventually (because they come last in the curriculum) surgeons complained — even railed — at the lack of anatomical knowledge in their latest students.

Yet nothing was done. It was not until the Harvard students became beginning doctors that they, too, complained. Their complaint was about *insecurity*; they just had *no idea what was beneath the skin*. And their complaints were made back to the Dean!

It was only then that something was done. But by then the anatomists had been largely fired, the bodies were not properly dissected, and visiting anatomists were imported (I was one of them; I saw the partially and poorly dissected bodies). It was a problem.

Thus, this component of undergraduate anatomy, anatomy for minor surgery, is widely misunderstood. A surgeon does need much more. But some anatomy **is necessary** for minor surgery or other simpler procedures of general practice.

Is Anatomy of Any Use for Doctors Who Will Never Cut?

Yes. Even more important than anatomy for major or minor surgery is anatomy for other specialties, for doctors who will never cut!

Thus, all doctors need to know, for example, how the local anatomy of special skin regions relates to edema: the swelling of the back of the hand and the top of the foot in the upright patient, the swelling around the eyes in the lying patient, or the swelling of the scrotum in the knees-up half-sitting patient (especially alarming to the patient in a cardiac bed). All relate to the special skin anatomies in those regions.

The same applies to haematomata (blood pools) in these same regions: on the back of the hand and the top of the foot, the 'black eye' that occurs not only from trauma, but as a result of the use of blood thinners, or the swelling and bruising of the scrotum after a hernia operation (so unexpected and so frightening if not previously explained to the patient).

Do we realize how important anatomy is for a large variety of clinical examinations? The opposite side test: pressing in the lower left aspect of the abdomen giving pain in the lower right aspect in appendicitis as gas is pushed backward along the colon. The obturator test: flexing and turning the right thigh inwards causing pain from a pelvic appendix where it lies on the obturator muscle. Chvostek's (naughty, naughty, using an eponym) test: tapping on the facial nerve (if you know where it is) elicits contraction of the facial muscles (if you know what they do) in hypocalcemia (if you understand what that is and why). Of course, given modern investigations, it may be thought such knowledge is not needed!

Do we understand that accuracy in observation and description in the clinic stems first from accuracy in simple observation and description in anatomy?

Do we realize, even, that anatomy is relevant to almost everything we do in medicine?

Yet Further: Is Not Anatomy Useful Simply for Medical Communication?

Do we not realize that anatomical terms and anatomical concepts are the vocabulary, syntax, and grammar of medicine, not just of anatomy? This is how doctors and other health professionals communicate not only with one another, but, more and more, with the medically educated public of today, especially patients and their relatives and carers.

For example, while pathology informs us about temporal arteritis, anatomy tells us what the temporal artery is. Neurology teaches about temporal lobe epilepsy, but anatomy tells us where the temporal lobe lies. Oncology teaches us how a breast cancer might give rise, sequentially, to a cough, back pain and headache, but anatomy reminds us of the anatomical pathways pursued by cancer cells from the breast, through the chest wall to the lung root, to the back of the chest, to the spinal column, and up the spinal canal to the skull cavity, to eventually, the brain.

My own general practitioner has an anatomical atlas and models on her shelves, as well as diagrams on her computer, so that she can explain more clearly to patients what is going on. And today's public wants the real thing, not some watered-down version.

Finally: How is Anatomy Learnt?

Even learning anatomy is widely misunderstood. It is so much more than the memorization of facts. Of course, memorization is an aid to learning in all disciplines.

Yet paradoxically, memorization was one of the reasons for eliminating anatomy. It seems like nothing needs to be memorized these days because Dr. Google can always 'look it up'. But the information in memorized texts, lists, pictures, notes, and

mnemonics, though all useful initially, disappear in short order, if
not used all the time. And if memory is replaced by 'the web', how
can one look up the anatomy if one has no initial understanding of
the science underlying it — its elements, relationships, development, functions and processes?

> *Pace memorization:* anatomy is only truly understood through its
> underlying science;
> *genetic mechanisms:* the initial blueprint of anatomy;
> *developmental processes:* building anatomy over a lifetime;
> *functional adaptation:* anatomy working;
> *experience and learning:* how anatomy is used;
> *medical applications:* when anatomy goes wrong; and even
> *evolutionary medicine:* anatomy as built and changed over myriads of
> lifetimes.

Anatomy can be memorized from textbooks, atlases, coloring
books, models, prosections and computers. These can, indeed, be
most useful, but may lead to **weak secondhand learning**.

Anatomy can be learnt from the body, of the living as well
as the dead, from fellow students, teachers, healthcare colleagues
and, naturally, of course, from patients. Anatomy can also — and
we often forget this — be learnt from ourselves. Our own bodies
are a 'cheat', but a legitimate useful cheat nevertheless, which we
can use in the library, the study carrel, the clinic, the bedside, and
even in the examination hall (I never said that!). Seeing, listening,
touching, speaking, discussing, using, and above all, questioning
the body all provide **powerful firsthand learning**.

Questioning is the first and final basis of learning; an interface
between the language of medicine and the language of life.

All this leads to a new problem for many of today's students.
In prior times, our students were often relatives of doctors or other
professionals and thus already possessed a medical flavor. They

usually had English as their first language. They had biological and classical backgrounds. They already 'knew' the meanings of most of the words.

In today's world, most students do not hail from medical families. Further, in today's world, many students are from language groups (e.g., Africa, Asia, Eastern Europe, the Middle East, and many others) far removed from English and most Western tongues. Even students whose language is English now lack the classics (Latin was compulsory in my day!) that used to be required for medicine.

Such students ask:

"Why do things have such complex names? If only we knew the meaning!"

They receive enlightenment (which they never forget) if it is explained to them that 'sartorius' is a muscle whose contraction produces the cross-legged sitting position as in an ancient Roman tailor (sartorius); hence the English phrase 'sartorial elegance', or 'tailored' elegance.

Another example comes from 'trapezius'. The two triangular trapezius muscles on the back of the shoulders taken together truly form a 'trapezium' (if we still have the mathematics to know what that is). The even older name for trapezius was 'cucullaris', like a cowl; the two muscles at their upper ends are shaped like the monk's cowl or 'scapula' (another medical term).

The teachers who understand the meanings of such words, and whose stories can enlighten the students, are also themselves almost extinct.

How My Anatomy Started

I started as an old-fashioned medical anatomist. I just escaped being a student in a medical anatomy course of *one thousand hours in two years* (the 'Edinburgh system')! I actually took the reduced (so by how much!) medical anatomy course of *six hundred hours in five terms* (the 'Birmingham system'). We dissected the entire human body and brain. We worked long out of hours. I even dissected an extra brain in the evenings in my bedroom! Most of us did; it was not illegal then. Or at least I don't think so! (Is there any defence from a statute of limitations?)

Later in Chicago, I taught anatomy in *two quarters* (a bit quick perhaps), and even later in Los Angeles, I taught anatomy in *one quarter*, still with entire body dissection. Think of that — the whole body in one quarter.

Most recently of all, I have been involved in courses where students do *not dissect at all*. Such courses are often not even labelled anatomy, but contain just enough anatomy, it is thought, to understand physiology. Our Dean allowed a very few students to elect dissection (but only of a single region of the body). Although 90% of the class wanted to do this, the Dean only accepted 40 lucky individuals. Even this has now gone!

These gradual reductions meant, paradoxically, that my own teaching became gradually better and better. The smaller the amount of teaching, the higher its quality!

But my own teaching really grew from helping someone else. How? It's an interesting story. I have written elsewhere of how Professor Zuckerman encouraged a young technician (Tom Spence) to take a degree in anatomical sciences. But I was the one who worked with him. I gave him one-on-one tuition in anatomy weekly for an entire year. It worked; he got the degree!

But though this helped Tom, it serendipitously did even more for me. I taught him by reinterpreting human anatomy through its scientific bases. Of course, at that time — the late fifties to early sixties of the twentieth century — that task was not easy.

The modern scientific underpinnings of anatomy — genetics, development, function, integration and evolution — just had not been taken far enough. I had to create the course for him. But it worked in spades!

Ever since that time, I have kept working on that idea.

Transplanting the Idea Across Half a World

The University of Chicago

Thus, I took this initial thinking from Birmingham anatomy (1950s and 1960s) in my move to University of Chicago anatomy (1960s and 1970s). Human anatomy was being transformed there under its then new Head, Ronald Singer, into a wider interest in vertebrate anatomy (even of some non-vertebrates!): their development, structure, function, and evolution. I was one of Singer's appointments in that transformation.

Thus, I became colored by the interests of the other staff, not just the medical anatomists, but the comparative anatomists, anthropologists, and evolutionary biologists who were already there: Singer himself, Stuart Altmann, James Hopson, Eric Lombard, Len Radinsky, Russ Tuttle, Leigh Van Valen and David Wake, among others. In addition were the other faculty in the cellular, molecular and neurobiology areas of the department.

This was strengthened by the Chicago research/teaching student cohort of those days: Gene Albrecht, Matt Cartmill, Rebecca German, Walter Greaves, Paul Heltne, Doug Lay, Betty Jean Manaster, Jane Peterson, Jim Shafland, Jack Stern, Tim Strickler, and Richard Wassersug, again among many others; graduate students who were to learn to teach as well as research.

Finally, these ideas were influenced by many visitors (some being pending appointments) that Singer and others attracted to the department: Fred Bookstein, George Lauder, La Barbera, later Neil Shubin (after my time, but a major influence through his book *Your Inner Fish*), and many others.

Though it was a human anatomy department, all these individuals were diving into the scientific underpinnings of anatomy in broad whole-organismal, developmental, functional, integrative, and evolutionary modes. (Some of these ideas were mirrored in that 1933 quotation and book of Zuckerman's, see earlier chapter.)

The University of Southern California

Though I later moved on to USC as Graduate Dean, I was also a professor in two departments, anatomy in the medical school and biology in the undergraduate college, and I was also a University Professor (with salary and research funds in the President's budget: one of only four in the university). Colleagues here included Gene Albrecht from Chicago (who had moved there independently of me), Fred Anapol, Brad Blood, Bruce Gelvin, Pete Lestrel, Joe Miller, and Sherry Gust, among others. Once again, we continued applying the underlying science to the teaching of anatomy.

Further, this was an especially seminal time for the medical students at USC. Many of them had started to realize that it might be important that they have a research/teaching side to their lives. Partly this was because of general interest. Partly, however, it was that they could see that medical practice could be leavened by research and teaching.

Thus, as Graduate Dean rather than Anatomy Professor, I was approached by a group of medical students (leaders Julie Graylow and Hugh Allen) who wanted to sample research in one or other of the laboratories around the medical school. I agreed to be director of a 'Medical Student Research Group'. This turned out to be highly successful as many of these students gave research papers at subsequent Western Medical Student Research Forums.

Next, I was approached by a group of medical students who already held undergraduate engineering degrees (led by medical student and engineer, Dan Zinder). They wanted to start an 'Engineers in Medicine Group' and Dan asked me to be its faculty director. I well remember a visit we made to a factory making internal lenses for the eye. We were amazed to realize that the rejection rate of these lenses was more than 98%, so tight were the specifications.

Finally, as a result of these endeavors (and probably partly because I had followed on Joe Ceithaml as director of the MD/PhD program in my last year in Chicago), I became the first director of a new 'MD/PhD program' at USC. This was a program in which the normal four years for an MD plus four years for a PhD could be collapsed into six years for the combined MD/PhD. It was done by using the elective time in the MD for some of the research time in the PhD. It was also done more quickly than usual because the students who opted for it (perhaps, better, who fought for it) were amongst the very best students.

The University of Western Australia

My final move to the University of Western Australia allowed further continuation of these ideas. Thus, I found that there already was a three/four year program at UWA that included non-medical undergraduate human anatomy (better labelled as human biology). The beginnings of the idea had been started by the Founding Professor of Anatomy, David Sinclair (and his short book, *Human Growth*, was still used). However, the broader human biology concept was very strongly supported by the next Established

Professor of Anatomy, David Allbrook, and it was mainly carried out through the masterminding of Dr. Len Freedman and further developed by all the academic staff, especially by Drs. Bill Blumer and Neville Bruce.

Of course, the human biology concept was opposed by many other departments worried about loss of students through the introduction of a new human biology discipline. There had been a similar reaction to the birth of human biology in the UK many years earlier. (I had been the Treasurer of the UK Society for the Study of Human Biology in the 1960s.)

The Perth department's name was changed to Anatomy and Human Biology, and when I arrived, the title of the Established Chair became Anatomy and Human Biology. I therefore became the first and also, as it turned out, the last holder of this Established Chair. (Established Chairs were to be later 'disestablished' and departments essentially eliminated, though in one of those reversals that tend to occur in academia, a School of Anatomy, Physiology and Human Biology within Human Science has been renamed!)

Thus, I found myself in an institution where these broader human biology ideas were already in full swing. It was a marriage made in heaven.

However, I did make a fundamental mistake! I met early with the Chairs of Physiology and Biochemistry and suggested that all three departments become a School of Medical Sciences (**I was not aware at that time that Professor Zuckerman himself had also made this mistake, at the beginning of his time in Birmingham**). I realized within moments of making this suggestion that it was a non-starter! The other departmental heads were dead against it, so the idea failed. Yet it was a shame.

We continued alone on the human biology route and we more than doubled in size. But physiology and biochemistry refused to go with us and fell by about half each! Human biology, of course, was not only in the faculty of medicine, but in the faculty of science, in university general education, and in higher education in the high schools of the state. This was not so for physiology and biochemistry. Our developments made the difference.

As in Birmingham, Chicago and Los Angeles, these ideas were further stimulated by a series of graduate students in the human biology area. These included, among others, the graduate students with whom I was particularly associated: Alanah Buck, Sara and Warren Flood, Dan Franklin, Vanessa Hayes, Jens Hirschberg, Robert Kidd, Algis Kuliukas, Nick Milne, Elizabeth Pollard, Pan Ruliang, Ken Wessen, and Willem de Winter. They, and of course many other students of the many other faculty, taught and researched in human biology.

So-Called Retirement

My final move has been into retirement. However, by a series of honorary post-retirement appointments over the last twenty-five years, and by the continued provision of an office, lab and research facilities by UWA, I have been enabled not only to continue with a fully funded research program, but also with a book teaching anatomy through its scientific bases.

Is Another Textbook of Human Anatomy Really Needed?

There are already a very large number of anatomy books. They range from huge tomes attempting to lay out most of human anatomy, to short summary books presenting the major facts in a pithy way. There are texts based upon anatomy from region to region (e.g., head and neck, thorax), to expositions that display anatomy in terms of systems (e.g., nervous, gastrointestinal, locomotor, etc). There are illustrated volumes from anatomy coloring books, to major atlases showing, through hundreds of (often confusing) leader lines, every anatomical detail. There are specialist books emphasizing the anatomy relevant to exemplar clinical problems and books of fully detailed clinical anatomy. There are even many ancillary texts showing specific parts of human anatomy (e.g., surface anatomy, imaging anatomy, anatomy for orthopaedics, anatomy for nurses, anatomy for artists, etc).

And almost all are available, even with animations, in various electronic and interactive guises. Also, almost without exception, these modes present human anatomy, in each of their different ways, as a roadmap of the human body to be memorized. As medical curricula have become increasingly crowded, the modern anatomical roadmap has become more and more limited. Today, the small books (and most of the other sources) used by medical students show only the 'motorways' and 'freeways'. The larger books have become references for the 'low ways' and 'byways' when required by the specialist.

The Scientific Bases of Human Anatomy: The Research/Teaching Nexus

After all this, why then did I think there was a need for another book (whether 'real' or 'electronic')?

Because I think that what is needed is a new system of human anatomy.

Because scientific understanding makes human anatomy, like any other science, derivative. It is to be handled, not memorized.

Because introducing underlying science makes human anatomy come alive in students' imaginations.

Because the scientific understanding of human anatomy is an important background not just to medicine per se, but also to many other disciplines such as:

human biology, functional anatomy, evolutionary biology, physical anthropology,
other basic medical life sciences such as physiology and biochemistry,
clinically related medical sciences: audiology, podiatry, nursing, sports studies, and
many zoological anatomies: primates, mammals, vertebrates, and others.

Because, most of all, major advances in several other sciences (such as genetics, developmental biology, molecular biology, growth, functional and behavioral biology, neurobiology and evolutionary biology) now provide exciting new insights into the how and the why of anatomy.

A New Developmental Biology

A new developmental biology is resulting from deeper knowledge of genes and other developmental molecules (Figure 4.1), and especially through recent developments in understanding genetics and developments from bioinformatics. When I was a student, there was a great gulf fixed between humans and most other creatures.

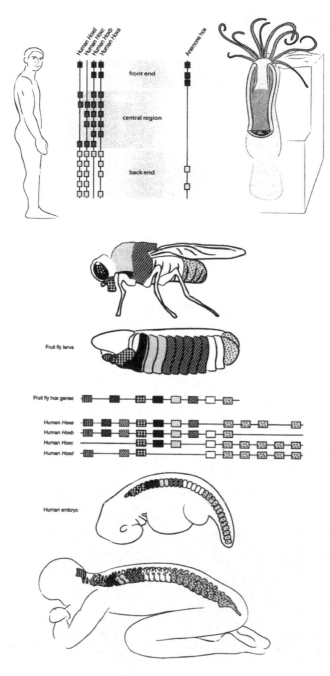

Figure 4.1: Top: a few Hox genes are shared between humans and sea anemones. Middle and bottom: many more Hox genes are shared between humans and fruit flies (redrawn after Shubin).

A New Comparative Morphology

A new comparative morphology has resulted from modern views of animal structure. The old comparative anatomy of my early years had become bogged down in the anatomy of *the* dogfish, *the* frog, *the* lizard, *the* pigeon, *the* rabbit. It had overlooked the fact that there are many kinds of cartilaginous fishes, amphibians, reptiles, birds and mammals, respectively.

This has now been corrected with a new burgeoning of comparative morphology that looks at diversity and complexity. As a result, it provides new evidence of underlying pattern for the anatomy of humans (Figure 4.2).

A New Functional Anatomy

A new functional anatomy is resulting from advances in bioengineering and biomathematics. It strengthens anatomical inferences, the main form of evidence in my earlier years (Figures 4.3 and 4.4). As a result, new ideas are emerging in testing and understanding the adaptations of anatomical structures.

Such new techniques help elucidate structure and function.

A New Wrinkle on the Brain

A new neurobiology is resulting from new non-invasive imaging techniques. Thus, the brain (Figure 4.5) can be seen through both the underlying molecular mechanisms for its development and the internal structures as it functions.

A New Evolutionary Biology

Finally, a new evolutionary biology has been evolving over many years now. It is a new, holistic, subject that joins the aforementioned advances as they culminate in evolution.

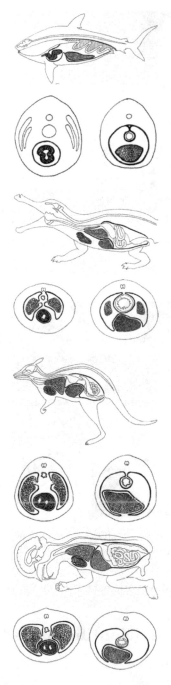

Figure 4.2: Longitudinal and cross sections of a cartilaginous fish, a reptile, a kangaroo, and a human (neonate) showing some anatomical similarities and differences across these species.

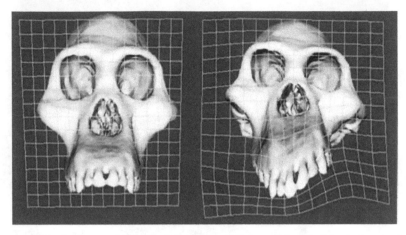

Figure 4.3:   Left: an unloaded monkey skull; right: a monkey skull loaded as in chewing on one side. The relationship between mechanics and architecture is clear (from Paul O'Higgins).

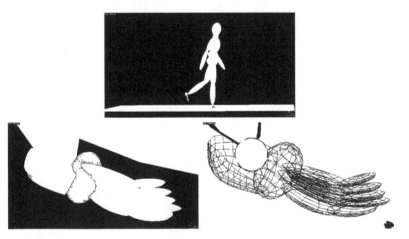

Figure 4.4:   Finite element analysis showing the human foot bearing loads in walking (thanks to Jonas Rubenstein and colleagues).

"All this," to modify Mayr's original quotation, *"is now human anatomy."*

Who Needs These Scientific Bases?

Medical Students?

The new system of human anatomy that I am describing **is not much use** to medical students in standard medical schools.

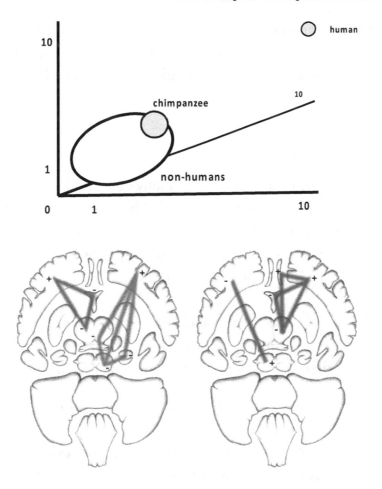

Figure 4.5: Human brains differ totally from other primates in terms of statistical analysis (above) that shows new internal connections (below). (See also later chapter.)

There is too much information, too much non-medical thinking; it is too far from immediate clinical needs, and there is no curricular room.

However, the medical curriculum in the USA, being postbaccalaureate in timing, allows topics like this new system to be played out in prior undergraduate programs. Many US universities and colleges have extensive collegiate premedical programmes. While most medical schools in Australia now also have four-year postgraduate programs, it has been at UWA in particular that a major human biology program, with human anatomy embedded within it, provides the basis for graduate medical and health-related qualifications.

Other Students!

But, this new system also appeals to many other students. They are students with no requirement for individual pieces of anatomical information until they need them for specific reports, term papers, study programs, research projects, grant proposals, dissertations and theses, and even, for beginning postdoctoral research and clinical applications.

If, however, they understand the scientific principles behind human anatomy, then when they come to need specific details, they can understand them rather than rely upon fading memory.

These include many other students specializing in many applied areas:

Students in various health-related areas who want an understanding of the anatomy of their patients,

Students in many human movement sciences (knowledge of specific anatomies is critical and enhanced by scientific approaches),

Students in biomechanics, bioengineering and medical engineering for whom, likewise, the science behind anatomy is critical,

And finally: students working in seemingly distant microstructural disciplines (that use microscopic and chemical methods) such as microanatomy, ultrastructural anatomy, physiology, pathology, biochemistry, and/or molecular biology. For these students, knowledge of human microstructures needs be placed in the context of human meso- and macrostructures.

In addition, some Australian universities are looking to new broad undergraduate experiences within which an understanding of the biology of humans may be a useful general component.

As a result, many undergraduates, far more than just the few who will next enter medical school, will find this new science-based human biology important.

From Dissection to Science

Anatomy traditionally involves the cutting of the body, whether 'real' (i.e., of the cadaver), 'pretended' (i.e., in a prosection, model, image or 3D-print), or even 'virtual' (i.e., in the computer). Personal dissection involves cutting and observing, usually from the outside in, from skin to bone. Prosected or modelled 'dissection' involves examining what someone else has cut or modelled. Virtual (computational) dissection may also be carried out by moving from the outside in, but interestingly, it can also be done in many other ways.

These other ways include:

'reverse dissecting' from the inside out, thus gradually clothing the bones,

'centripetal dissecting' from the center to periphery, following spiderweb-like systems (nerves, lymphatics, blood vessels),

'local dissecting' where systems (nerves, blood vessels, glands, organs) may be conflated,

'dendritic' dissection following the tree-like pathways of development and growth, or

'island' dissection following islands of related structures such as the scattered endocrine glands, scattered lymph nodes, or even, clinically, scattered cancer metastases.

Such approaches provide new and improved roadmaps of the body. However, without further exposition, they do not easily provide scientific understanding. In fact, they often do the opposite, especially through their testing mechanisms. The testing mechanisms tend to present the learning of human anatomy as 'the naming of the parts'. Indeed, 'the naming of the parts' is often how anatomy is taught and, even more often, how it is learned.

I thought this was my idea, but it was a WA colleague, Jan Meyer, who drew my attention to a little poem titled *The Naming of Parts*. It was about the anatomy of guns, but it might as well have been about the anatomy of bodies:

> *To-day we have naming of parts.*
> *Yesterday, we had daily cleaning.*
> *To-morrow, we shall have firing.*
> *But to-day, we have naming of parts.*

The old approaches to anatomy involved naming of parts: large numbers of small details. They were often reinforced through the use of mnemonics, eponyms, acronyms and even jokes (usually crude and today, politically unacceptable). They can be helpful in the short term for examinations that emphasize the reproduction of facts and names. This kind of information does not last in the long term, **and it is as boring as hell**.

As an example, my wife reintroduced me to modern medical examinations. She volunteers in the US Education Advisory Service in the US Consulate in Perth. She brought home the practice disc (USMLE) used by Australian doctors wanting to go to the USA and insisted that I take it. I resisted, but after several days she wore me down. So, I started with surgical anatomy. Though I am no surgeon, as an anatomist I got the first six questions right, so I was bored and gave up.

The next section was molecular medicine. Now, molecular medicine had not been invented in 1960 when I was last in practice. The ultrastructure of the cell was poorly known then. There was little medical genetics. The electron microscope had not long been invented. Cell biology was new. I took the first cell biology course in Birmingham, which comprised just five lectures!

Yet I obtained 37.5 out of 50 marks in that USMLE test of molecular medicine. What does this mean, and how did I do it? Of course, it's the stupidity of multiple choice examinations. I didn't know the correct answer to any individual molecular question, but I knew just enough science and medicine to divine the answers that were wrong!

It has well been documented how memorization without understanding (except when memorized at mother's knee) disappears so easily. It is indeed one of the reasons why many practicing professionals, especially some in the non-cutting specialities, remembering that hateful memorizing activity as students, resent anatomy. This reaction in many current medical professionals is yet another of the many factors underlying the elimination of anatomy.

Yet other practicing professionals feel the opposite. They recognize the enjoyment that they had in anatomy and the lifelong friendships they made there. It was the only time in the old medical curricula where the same small group of students knew, helped and worked with one another and the same teachers for a whole year (even a whole two years in the most ancient of days!). In the new medical curriculum, this academic camaraderie is now lost. In fact, today, no part of medical education lasts long enough to provide such student/staff interaction.

The New System of Anatomy

The method I (and of course, also many others) have developed over the years, in contrast to 'the naming of the parts', is a holistic integrative approach to human structure. It involves understanding that the structural details of the human body are the end results of a series of biological processes.

These processes produce anatomical pattern due to:

blue prints of body building from genes and related molecules in *beginning time*,
tool kits for change in growth and differentiation over *developmental time*,
comparisons of different forms living at the *same time*,
adaptations to biological, chemical and physical factors during *functional time*,
interactions between body and brain, brain and body, through *integrative time*, and
innovation in structures resulting from evolution in *deep time*.

This way of approaching the anatomy of the body starts at the opposite end from the traditional. Instead of memorizing the details of the body as dissected, prosected, demonstrated or even studied electronically in a geographic manner, the principles of body construction can be looked at from their beginnings, whether those beginnings are genetic, developmental, adaptive, comparative, integrative or evolutionary.

I once was involved in a study of the anatomy of ships (see another chapter). What shipwright would try to understand how to build a ship by taking it to pieces, rivet by rivet?

Shipwrights know how a ship is built starting from, and following, plans (an anatomist sees these plans as heredity and development). Shipwrights improve ships by assessing what features of the ship worked last time (an anatomist sees adaptation to function). Shipwrights understand the comparisons of ships built for different purposes (an anatomist uses comparison of creatures with different lifestyles). Shipwrights realize the importance of communication mechanisms in ships, so enormously elaborated in these days of electronics and computers (an anatomist sees communication and integration between body and brain). Shipwrights recognize that the changes in shipbuilding techniques over the generations of shipbuilders provide an archive of shipbuilding (an anatomist sees the archive of evolution, even if it is incomplete).

These are most useful bases from which to understand the anatomy of ships and the way they work. So, too, it is for the anatomy of the body.

Nevertheless, this does not mean that dissections and details are not important. An archaeological shipwright may need to take the 'remains' of a 'fossil' ship to pieces for comparison with the 'anatomies' of 'living' ships in order to understand novel or unexpected ways in which shipwrights of the past thought and worked. They might even, then, rebuild 'fossil' ships from the extant fragments that they find. A palaeontologist may, likewise, need to use pieces of fossils for rebuilding (reconstructing) the fossil species for comparison with the anatomies of living human relatives. Reconstruction is a *sine qua non* not only for the marine archaeologist, but for the anatomist and anthropologist. Except that we often get it so wrong.

Thus, some of these ideas are not as new as I may be appearing to suggest.

Many very old texts attempted these approaches, but were limited by what little was then known. Today, the excitement of new concepts cries out to illuminate human anatomy.

But where, the student, the clinician, and the examiner, may ask, in such a system is the classical anatomical information, such as the 'triangles of the neck', the 'back of the abdomen', the 'axilla', or even, the 'maze of blood vessels around the knee'? The answer is that they are not directly in this new system! They can already be found, in greater or lesser detail, in any of many large or small anatomy texts.

Anatomical information does appear in this new approach, of course, but only from the viewpoint of the underlying sciences. It is in a largely new guise. Yet is it really the case that this new approach has not been attempted before?

In fact, even long before Darwin's time, many individuals tried to use scientific underpinnings as ways of understanding human structure.

Apart from the books of the Ancients and the Renaissance, a more recent early book was Todd and Bowman's *Physiological Anatomy of Man* (1845). It was specifically aimed at both students and practitioners of medicine and surgery. This was at a time when it was clearly understood that anatomy, physiology, medicine and surgery all went together! Another was the use of vertebrate anatomy by Wiedersheim (1892) to illuminate a specifically human anatomy. Yet another that also unashamedly used this approach was Sir Arthur Keith's *Human Embryology and Morphology* just after the turn of the century (1902). So how new is it really?

There have also been many later 20th century books that contained this approach. They include, for example, J. Z. Young's two farsighted books: *Life of Mammals* (1966) and *Life of Vertebrates* (1981). Likewise, in a different vein and yet also employing elements of this approach, is Milton Hildebrand's wonderful *Analysis of Vertebrate Structure* (1974). These, and others, are excellent books and still, in my opinion, very useful. But because they were originally written many years ago, they do not include the mass of new genetic, developmental, comparative, functional, integrative and evolutionary information.

Furthermore, unlike the earlier essays by Todd and Bowman, Wiedersheim, and Keith, these later books were not aimed at human anatomy. They usually only include humans as a minor example of another mammal, another tetrapod, another vertebrate, etc. To be very fair, they were not aimed at understanding humans in the first place.

Further, approaches like those suggested here also exist in a number of excellent 'evo-devo' texts published even more recently (across the century divide). These, naturally, do include the new scientific information. Indeed, these books, and the primary literature on which they are based, have been most important to me in describing some of the underlying concepts. They include, among many, for example, B. K. Hall's *Evolutionary and Developmental Biology* (1999) and R. M. Twyman's *Developmental Biology* (2001). Again, however, these books are primarily aimed at explicating the evolutionary and developmental anatomy of many forms: primates, mammals, tetrapods, vertebrates, and so on. Again, therefore, their thrust is not human anatomy specifically. The human anatomy is secondary, just another animal in the broader picture.

Yet other useful books include primary human embryology and developmental biology texts. W. J. Larson's *Human Embryology* (1993 and later editions) and B. M. Carlson's *Human Embryology and Developmental Biology* (2004) figure among these. They are excellent texts. But while they provide many important and fascinating linking materials from other species, they are fully aimed at humans even if they are separate from human anatomy *per se*.

The final set of books that use elements of the approach adopted here are genuinely human anatomy books. They include Matt Cartmill, Bill Hylander and Jim Shafland's *Human Structure*

(1987) and Jack Stern's *Essentials of Gross Anatomy* (1988), among a number of others.

The first of these two books (Cartmill, *et al.*) provides considerable explanatory information from developmental, functional and evolutionary biology. However, because it was written many years ago, it does not include the more recent linking material. Further, its organization is still largely based on the traditional anatomical regions.

The second of these two books (Stern) is an even more standard human anatomy text for medical students. Yet it, too, integrates much information about developmental, comparative and functional aspects of human anatomy. For example, in one place, Stern gives an excellent description of the changes in limb form during evolution, common in vertebrate anatomy texts, unusual in human anatomy texts.

Finally, there is a beautiful book by Neil Shubin. This book, *Your Inner Fish*, is a journey into the 3.5 billion-year history of the human body. It provides vignettes on the long, long, journey to human anatomy, rather than on the final human anatomy itself. It is a wonderful introduction to human anatomy and the science behind human anatomy.

Let me emphasize, I do not criticize any of these texts; I owe much to them and to others not cited.

The Research/Teaching Nexus Idea: My Teaching Hopes

A first hope is that this new system will introduce the student to the use of the scientific underpinnings of human anatomy as a major rationale for understanding it.

A second hope is that the student will realize that this system cannot cover everything in anatomy in an equal manner. It certainly cannot capture the whole of human anatomy. Why these hopes?

One answer is that it is my aim to introduce students to principles in some parts, while adding to their learning by leaving it to them to work out the extensions of the principles in other parts. In other words, I want the students to *build on the story!*

A second answer is that the principles have not yet been equally and fully worked out in all areas. I myself have worked in only a few areas. Some of my ideas may well turn out to be wrong (see other chapters)! In other words, I want students to see that I don't know the full story, that no one ever will, and that, therefore, *there are more questions to be asked!*

A third answer is that the complete understanding and then integration of all these basic sciences and their application to human anatomy is too much to ask of any single author, certainly of this author. In other words, *this is only an idea in progress!*

A final and most important answer is the hope that through these questions and answers, some right and some wrong, students will come to realize the many other interesting questions that they can ask in their own research, whether expressed as simple curiosity, term papers, undergraduate honors projects, practical applications, postgraduate theses and dissertations, or even later, academic studies, papers and books, as the students, in turn, progress. In other words, I want them to be stirred into undertaking their own research endeavors, finding their own answers, *and most of all asking their own new questions, in their own futures.*

In this context, I have never forgotten the words of one young academic when I was asked to review the status of a particular anatomy department. This was a young man, absolutely fascinated by anatomy, outgoing to his students, deeply concerned with teaching as well as he could, and, I could see, a teacher very much liked by his students. I asked during the interview:

"What about your research?"
He told me.

Later at the kind of social occasion that also occurs in such situations, I met him again over drinks. I repeated my question:
"Tell me more about your research in human anatomy."
"Well,"
he said, honestly,
"to tell you the truth I am not very interested in my research. I do it because I know I have to publish for my career. I do it because it gives me something to tell people like you when you come around."
"So, why are you so interested in teaching human anatomy?" I asked.
"Because I love the structure of human anatomy,"
he said,
"because I love how complete it is,"
"because I love to present this completed structure to the students,"
"because I love the fact that it is so complete,"
he continued,
"because there are no more questions to be asked!"

No matter how good and attractive this teacher is to his students, if he leaves them with the notion that his subject is complete, that there are no more questions to be asked, then I aver that he is a very bad teacher indeed.

> It is my fervent desire that this new system should show how the new work in other disciplines can provide new questions for anatomy.
> It is my fervent desire, too, that this new system will also present new questions for other disciplines.
> It is my final fervent desire that new questions will come thick and fast to my students.

5 First Practice: The Teaching/Research/Practice Triad

As it became clear to me that my life was going to be in basic medical research, I also already knew this would include teaching basic medical sciences to medical (and other) students. Further, although I knew I would never practice medicine as a career, I dearly wanted my research and teaching to be leavened by interests in, knowledge of, and applications to clinical medicine. I therefore set out to make sure that I had at least a 'smidgen' of clinical practice.

So, after qualifying in medicine, I spent time doing general medicine and surgery, and clinical rotations in ear, nose and throat, eyes, skins, obstetrics and gynaecology, and even some locums in general practice.

This has paid off in spades, especially in more recent times, and particularly in the last few decades, where anatomy teachers, unless old, are very likely to be neither medically qualified nor have any firsthand medical experience. The students always seemed to appreciate the flavor of this brand of anatomy for medicine. It could only be superficial, but I hoped it would be enough for me to provide clinical links.

It was only later that I realized the many unexpected research benefits that can grow from a continuing interest in clinical practice.

Beginning Clinical Experiences

Accordingly, then, after the MB/ChB degree, I did the regulation hospital jobs in general medicine and general surgery to be registered as a medical practitioner. I also taught in various aspects of medicine in several clinical departments, and even had just a 'lick' of general practice.

One reason I did more practice was a desire to remain totipotential for a little while longer. A second was to get, if I could, top medical jobs, with references from top academic clinicians! A third was the fact that I enjoyed clinical medicine and was not yet ready to give it up. A fourth reason was the realization that if I entered research, I likely would also be teaching medical students, and I felt that some experience of real practice, even if only a little, would be invaluable for my teaching.

A fifth and final reason, though I did not know it at the time, was that my small knowledge of clinical medicine was to lead me, serendipitously, to some fascinating investigations that a pure anatomist (or a pure physician) might never have recognized.

Accordingly, I first took up house jobs (called internships today) at the Queen Elizabeth Hospital, Birmingham, the premier teaching hospital in that part of England. At that time, it was the most up-to-date teaching hospital in England (completed just before the war). It produced, from among its various doctors over subsequent years, the Presidents of several of the Royal Colleges.

Fifty years after my time, the QE real estate had become rather rundown. But it has now been replaced with a magnificent new hospital (still called the Queen Elizabeth Hospital; no changing of the name!).

I worked first in General Medicine with Drs Carey Smallwood and Clifford (the 'Hawk') Hawkins. Carey did wonders for my abilities in phlebotomy. In those days, the medical students took all the 'bloods'. But in my year, the students complained that they had too many. So, Carey decreed that I, as the houseman, should take them all. I was so cross. But I became good at it! And I also ordered fewer. *This might have been Carey's way of telling me I ordered too many!*

The Hawk gave me a book for Christmas; not Stephen Potter's *One-Upmanship*, but his later *Supermanship. The Hawk, too, may have been telling me something!*

I clearly remember one incident during this job, when I had three patients in a row with different types of asthma. I had read all about asthma and was deeply into the condition, but the fourth patient was a heart attack. I was so cross. I was into asthma; the heart attack was a distraction. *Not a good attitude for a doctor!*

And I equally clearly remember something else from this time. I used thalidomide, a wonderful drug for helping to get old people off to sleep at night. Of course, it was only later that it was realized that thalidomide caused problems in pregnancy! Thank goodness I was doing general medicine; all my patients were old and hence not facing pregnancy risks!

Next was general surgery with Professor Stammers and his senior registrar, Geoff Slaney (later a President of the Royal College of Surgeons of England). Professor Stammers was originally a neurosurgeon but, unusually (perhaps because of the war), had become a general surgeon.

Thus, Prof. Stammers now did mastectomies for breast cancers and gastrojejunostomies for gut ulcers. Of course, radiation treatment for cancers was only just coming in, while *Helicobacter pylori* as a cause of ulcers was in the far future (for which Barry Marshal and Robin Warren of the University of Western Australia got the Nobel Prize)!

Doing Stammer's surgical job also required me to work in orthopedics with Mr. Tom Donovan. He was old, grey and pretty crusty. Professor Stammers had determined that the only way Donovan would get a house surgeon was if he shared his own house surgeon with him.

I have never forgotten my first orthopaedic operation. It was my first day, which meant, of course, that I had not seen the patient before. The first I saw of the patient were his two feet.
"Right,"
said Tom Donovan,
"you take this foot, I'll take the other!"
It was a case of bilateral bunions. I had never seen the operation, nor did I even know its principle. When Tom made a curved incision in the patient's foot, I made the mirror image incision in mine. What he did, I copied in reverse. He was practiced and fast; I was inexperienced and slow. I got further and further behind. I had the additional stress of remembering the sequence of actions. At last the operation ended; everyone seemed satisfied!

It happened that I was not expected to attend the outpatient clinic afterwards. Therefore, I never knew whether my side might not have been better than his!

I also remember assisting at another of Donovan's operations to remove a plate from a bone that had become infected and not healed. During the op, a small screw fell into the bottom of the deep wound; it was hidden by the slow welling up of blood. One did not, of course, put one's hand into the wound; we were using the 'no touch technique'. So, we prodded around in the pool of blood with long forceps trying to find the screw. Donovan was getting more and more irritated. Geoff Slaney (his senior registrar) was equally fed up.

After about twenty minutes, Donovan turned his head so that the theater sister could wipe the sweat out of his eyes. Quick as a flash, Slaney had his hand into the wound, found the screw, put it into the forceps with his fingers, and exclaimed,

"Look, I've got it!"

There was one particular occasion on which I had to assist at the General Hospital in Birmingham. It was a simple appendicectomy. The surgeon was very tall; the theater sister was very small; the operating table was surrounded by benches for her to stand on. Of course, we were all masked and capped. The only part of my face that the surgeon could see were my eyes.

At the critical moment of the operation, he held up this swollen, purple and yellow, pus-filled horror of an appendix.
"Don't look at my work like that, my boy,"
he looked at me and said,
"that's the kind of look you reserve for dogs copulating in the street!"
Could he really see my face behind my mask?

I enjoyed all this very much. But one of the most important things I learnt was how to organize my time when, in those days, there could be near eighty hours of work a week, and only for 5 pounds sterling! I even kept a diary, but only for two weeks; there was no time! While it was not clever and actually rather dangerous, that was the way it was in those days, and to some degree is still today.

Pharmacology and Therapeutics

My first experience in teaching in the clinical arena was in pharmacology and therapeutics.

Even as a student, I was deputed to teach about drugs acting on the heart and blood vessels, especially those used in heart failure. In those days, treatment of heart failure included diuretics. But I started it by telling the students about the ancient way of removing fluid from swollen limbs: Southey Tubes (Figures 5.1 and 5.2).

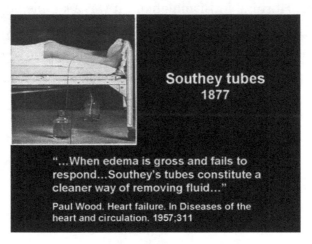

Figure 5.1: Southey Tubes, 1877.

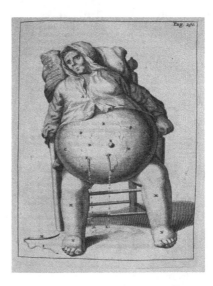

Figure 5.2: Tubes even before Southey: Leiden, 1694.

Next, I moved on to the then current methods of treating oedema: diuretic drugs like acetazolamide, the mercurials, and so on (there weren't too many in those days).

But I always tried to introduce the students to new, experimental (as they were at the time) drugs just so that they would be prepared to look for improvements. One such drug was spironolactone, which was at that point not used in practice, and I never knew that one day spironolactone would truly enter the medical kit-bag. Nor did I realize that I myself would depend upon it as a prophylactic for the 'cerebral oedema' of my own 'high altitude sickness' later. Spironolactone (rather than acetazolamide) was the drug preferred by the Royal Australian Airforce at that time.

I totally 'failed' in the teaching of antibiotics in the following sense: I had emphasized

that patients should take the whole course (and not stop when symptoms disappeared),
that doctors should use antibiotics sparingly (and not apply them to every snuffle),
and that both the patients' demands for the then new miracle drugs for everything, and the many
pharmaceutical companies demands' for overprescribing, must be resisted, but perhaps these weren't emphasized hard enough.

Much antibiotic resistance today may be laid at the door of, among other things, my failure (and that of many other teachers of my generation) to get such ideas across!

Bites at General Practice

I also undertook some 'locum tenens' appointments in general practice. Partly it was for the money, I must admit; young doctors were very poor in those days (and they still are today). But I undertook them just as much to expand my beginning clinical practice experience.

During one locum, I worked alongside an experienced general practitioner (I was taking the place of his partner). Though I was not experienced, I actually saw about 34 patients in about two and a half hours! On average, five minutes each! I was horrified.

But I was far more horrified to find that my more experienced colleague saw about 50 patients in the same time! I cannot believe that this is good medicine even though he was a very good GP, and the patients had already been 'weeded out' by a very competent nurse/receptionist. It was the system that was horrifying!

I also did a *locum tenens* for another general practice, one with a 'lockup clinic'. That is, the main practice had a subsidiary clinic at another address that was locked. Given a key, I would open it up, do the clinic, and lock it again!

It was also known as a 'one-syringe clinic'. There really was only one syringe that had to be boiled up for each patient! There was also only one needle. One had to ream out the dried blood, resharpen the needle, and sterilize it for reuse. Nothing disposable in those days!

And so, of course, there was no nurse! An evening arrived when three teenage girls came to the clinic. They had heard that there was a doctor with a beard. This giggling group wanted to see him as a threesome! In a lock-up clinic with no chaperone — I got rid of them in a flash!

Other Teaching: Insurance, Police, Ambulance, Nurses

Again, because Eleanor and I were poor, I looked for other sources of income. They readily came. I was paid to teach 'anatomy, physiology and common medical conditions' to insurance students! This was a real challenge — to get those students excited when all they saw was simply the rote learning of the meanings of a lot of big words. *It was a subject they hated!* So, I put a lot of effort into telling them the stories behind the big words, in making the 'big words' sing. This totally turned the course around and they enjoyed every minute of it. It also gave me a lot of experience in explaining medicine to regular folks. This experience was to serve me well when, much later, I gave lectures on science and medicine to the general public. I even taught emergency medicine to the police and the St. John's Ambulance Brigade. In those days, there was no external heart massage, no defibrillator, and it was even before the days of the Heimlich maneuver (Figure 5.3) for dislodging an object stuck in the throat (now not recommended).

I well remember trying to get the emergency medicine students to estimate (approximately) the amount of blood that might be lost in an accident. I splashed a cup of milk (milk shows up

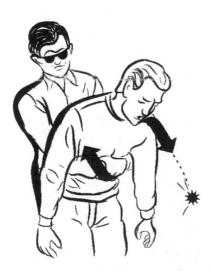

Figure 5.3: The Heimlich maneuver (no longer recommended).

well on a black slate floor), followed by a whole bottle of milk, in order to show just how much surface area these different volumes can cover. And I pointed out to them just how much blood could be hidden within the chest, within the belly, even within a thigh, when internal bleeding has occurred. And when a baby haemorrhages, even a very small blood loss may be critical!

I even tutored nursing students. Once again, the problem was that they thought learning anatomy was a feat of memory. It always gave me great pleasure to see the wonderment in their eyes when they realized that it was not based on memory but derivative! If one understands the underlying science, the anatomy comes easily. And in turn, there was much that I learnt from nurses that is never taught by doctors, like a man wiggling his toes to obviate the discomfort of a first cystoscopy!

I once even acted as 'the doctor' at the ringside in amateur boxing for 12 year-olds (something I think of as abominable today). I discovered how vicious parents can be! Came the moment when blood was spilt from a bloody nose, I immediately stopped the fight. I thought the parents were going to lynch me; I never did it again (attend at a boxing match, I mean)!

Because I taught elements of emergency medicine to the local St. John's Ambulance Brigade, I had many friends among them. I was permitted to ride with the ambulance, and to hang out of the window, ringing the bell, as we proceeded through the streets. No sirens in those days!

When on one occasion I was hauled before a court through a minor car accident (in which, luckily, no one was hurt), I said, as an academic person would:
"I *thought* the lights were green."
The other individual, being a 'real person', said:

"The lights *were* green."

I had a string of my students, nurses, St. John's ambulance workers, and even policemen, as 'character witnesses'. It did no good; I got the 'hanging judge' — fine: ten pounds!

Specialty Rotations, Especially Psychiatry

I also did some clinical rotations that gave me a few weeks each of ear, nose and throat, eyes, skins, obstetrics, psychiatry, and so on. This was a way to get a quick view of a number of subjects, again providing me with a little breadth that, subsequently, proved most useful for medical student teaching.

I am not sure I approve of what I learnt in the dermatology clinic. If the lesions are wet, apply a drying agent; if dry, a wetting agent, and for all else apply tar! And I was taught the old saw: do dermatology and your patients never die, *but neither do they get better!*

I have especially never forgotten my psychiatric experiences. One could do a few Saturday mornings in a local psychiatric clinic or a fortnight in residence at a very large psychiatric hospital. I thought I would learn very little in the morning clinics, so I opted for residence.

The hospital was deep in the beautiful Warwickshire countryside. As I did not, at that point, drive, Eleanor, with whom I was not, at that point, married, drove me there. We came in through a magnificent gatehouse, up a winding drive, through what looked like a broad park with stands of trees, undulating lawns, flower beds and bushes, and lots of benches sprinkled around the grounds. It was a delicious afternoon: the sun was shining and people were scattered around on the benches; idyllic!

Then, as happens so often in England, came a small, quick, dark cloud. As it started to rain, we quickly realized where we were as the people remained seated on the park benches in the rain! White-clothed workers ran out from the buildings to take the 'sittees' back inside. That time gave me experiences of psychiatry, especially emergency psychiatry, which I would never have received in a few hours of outpatient clinics.

There was one case that I especially remember. A woman was brought in to the casualty (emergency) department by the local police. She had been found wandering in a local village in her night clothes. She presented as showing a 'fugue', a word describing a mental state of flight, like the flight of instruments in a 'musical fugue'. Initial diagnoses were all, of course, psychiatric; after all, she had been brought to a psychiatric hospital! I worked hard on the work-up.

I found a lump in her breast, and she also had a cough and backache. X-rays showed shadows inside the chest just under the breast bone. Did these spread from the breast? There were more shadows at the lung root (perhaps, hence, the cough), as well as at the back of the lungs lying against and into the bodies of the vertebrae (perhaps, hence, the backache).

Further, in this position at the back of the chest, the shadows (secondary spread from the breast?) would be extremely close, perhaps only a millimeter or so, to the sleeve-like prolongation of the membranes that extend from the spinal cord along the spinal nerves as they emerge from the spine.

Once in the cerebrospinal fluid contained in this membrane, cancer cells could float headwards, pass into the skull and seed out, possibly, in the brain, perhaps even the temporal lobe. Hence, possibly, the fugue! Such beautiful anatomical 'raisons d'êtres' for an apparently psychiatric case!

I remember another case that completely took me in. A man with military bearing was not complaining of anything, but here he was, in a mental hospital. I was told to take a history; there seemed to be nothing obvious. I wondered: "Why was he here?"

So, I went into his life history in detail. It was fascinating; I listened to him for about half an hour. A real raconteur!

He had been in the Middle East during the second world war and out of this had arisen his later involvement in the oil industry. He had become fairly high up in a particular oil company.

A question about his war experiences elicited a series of escapades in arms. He had never been captured, but had been in the desert 'with Monty'. He had been mentioned in dispatches! Then I discovered that he had been decorated. A few more questions led to him revealing that he had received the Victoria Cross! Yet more questions, and he had a bar to his Victoria Cross!!

Finally, he admitted to 40 Victoria Crosses!!!

The early part of his story was so believable. But as I pressed him with questions, his story became more and more unbelievable. This was a sign of 'delusions of grandeur'; in his case a late effect of syphilis, and possibly a late effect of the war!

Some of my cases did not come from practice. I stopped at a garage, at which I was known, to get petrol.
"Hey Doc,"
said one of the attendants,
"this old guy has just fallen off his bicycle. Could you have a look at him?"
So, I did.

I described him as 'an old man of 65'. Today I would describe him as a young man of 65! He had indeed just fallen off his bicycle but had hobbled into the filling station, so I took a history.

Among other things, I asked him if it hurt when he walked.

"Yes," but he said he felt a bit bruised. Indeed, he was able to walk up and down, which he demonstrated to me. However, as I watched him, I realized his right foot was turned outwards by nearly 90 degrees.

"Has your foot always been turned out like that?"

I asked.

He looked surprised. Apparently, no one had ever asked him that question before!

"Yes," he said "all my life."

One must listen to patients, but in some cases, one must take what they say with a grain of salt!

So, I was suspicious, and sent him to hospital. I was so lucky.

A radiograph showed that he had fractured the neck of his right femur; the thigh muscles had turned the lower thigh outwards, hence his foot turned outward. But the rest of the fall must have driven the neck of the femur back into the shaft in the new position so that continuity was restored, but with the leg rotated. Hence, with only a little pain, he could still walk, but with his foot pointing out!

At first, these early professional experiences fascinated me in their own right. I have often wondered what would have happened to me if I had taken the direction of clinical practice alone. Certainly, I found an acute excitement in practice, and I enjoyed the contacts that I had with patients, their relatives, and colleagues of many kinds. Of course, other doctors, especially more senior doctors, were obviously important. But in particular, the experienced nurses and laboratory technicians, and even the mortuary attendants and the hall porter, were also very important in my education as a young doctor.

For example, I always attended whenever a nurse asked me to see a patient, even if they were a little yellow (a QE hospital beginning nurse), and even in the middle of the night. Sometimes it was indeed to help a sick patient, sometimes to reassure an anxious nurse, but often to cover my own worries and inexperience. All were important. And I was taught such a lot by the nurses, often things that the doctors never taught.

And whenever I ordered a clinical test that I had not ordered before, I always went down to the laboratory (why were the labs almost always underground in those days) and have the technician explain to me how it was done and what it was all about. I learnt so much from the laboratory workers, and they were always delighted that a 'young doctor' came to see them instead of just sending down a peremptory request form. And of course, whenever I needed something in a genuine hurry, these technicians would happily oblige because they knew me.

It was especially important to be familiar with the dispensary. I had one patient with a rapidly enlarged liver. Rapid enlargement stretches the liver capsule, causing pain. He complained and complained about the pain, but no medication seemed to resolve it. So, my consultant (Dr. Oscar Brenner) ordered 'leeches'! That was news to me. Of course, I had to get the leeches, but where do you get them? It turned out to be the dispensary. There they were, under a bell jar. Put mustard on their tails to empty their stomachs (causes vomiting), and place the leeches on the patient around the liver region. It worked! Or at least, he stopped complaining!

A different kind of experience was my first dying patient. I saw her several times over my six-month job. She was about nineteen years old; almost my age. She was so beautiful, but so thin and ethereal, having been inflicted with Hodgkin's disease.

The treatment in those days was blood transfusions. I had to give them, but by then she had almost no accessible veins left, so getting a needle in was very difficult.

Such beginning clinical experiences could not have been a better preparation for teaching medical students. This became evident in spades when I came to teach in the United States and Australia where anatomy teachers so rarely have medical degrees. The students loved my mixture of scientific knowledge, medical insights, clinical anecdotes.

So, I really enjoyed my early clinical experiences. However, in addition to enlivening my teaching, I came to realize that these various early professional experiences took me into new research projects that I would never otherwise have recognized. There is a tripartite relationship between teaching, research and practice. We never know how an obvious thing for an obvious purpose gives an unexpected thing for an unexpected purpose!

The Triad Idea: Teaching, Research, Practice

Thus, notwithstanding the excitement of clinical work, I was determined to return to research. Prof. Stammers himself was disappointed. He wanted me to enter surgery, but he nevertheless strongly supported my decision for research. And when, many years later, I returned to Birmingham to receive a DSc (in science and engineering, not medicine), he came to the degree ceremony!

I imagine most people understand that teaching throws up questions for research, and that research, if we will let it, can greatly change teaching. I have often documented this bipartite relationship, the research-teaching nexus. Unfortunately, it is often ignored by medical educators, managers and bureaucrats. It has certainly been denigrated by administrators and politicians.

It seems cheaper to separate teaching from research, to employ to teach only those who do no research, and vice versa!

Thus, while I continued my medical training as a clinical medical student and later a junior doctor, I also continued with my original research in my spare time. Some of this is described in the previous chapter. What spare time does a clinical medical student, a beginning doctor, have?

However, in those early years as an incredibly busy young doctor, I was much less aware of another very important relationship: a 'triad' that also includes the professional relationship of practice. Perhaps, while recognizing intellectually that there would be a triple relationship between teaching, research and practice, I was too busy to understand, too rushed to try, and too tired to think.

Yet even though I'm now no longer practicing, I have kept theoretical contact with clinical medicine. Long after I left clinical medicine, I continued reading the medical textbooks — Cecil and Loeb (medicine) and Big Anderson (pathology) were my favorites. Today, Dr. Google is sometimes an excellent, even if sometimes a lying, mentor! I have continually tried to understand new finds in medicine as they have come along.

As I did so, I became aware that, enjoyable as teaching and practice were, there was, for me, a different, deeper, excitement in research. It was at this point that I realized the importance of the triad teaching/research/practice relationship! Life, however, is not a controlled experiment; we can never know where different choices may take us.

A first such example involves bone and bones. Thus, as a medical student, yet at the same time doing research on the skeletons of monkeys and apes, I had an abiding interest in all aspects of bone and bones.

So, I especially read everything I could about bones. This included reading about the problems of osteoporosis and rickets, about functionally unusual (to me) bones such as the middle ear bones, about occasional bone variants like 'ectopic' bones, bones in curious places like tendons (rider's bone), the bladder wall, and the heart (in large animals, the *os cordis*), other extra (supernumerary) bones (e.g., the *os centrale*, found rarely in the wrist of humans but always in the wrists of apes), and even about the many problems of human bone growth including the various gigantisms and dwarfisms. I was delighted when a technician, who had been mounting an orang utan skeleton for display, came to me with a sheepish look on his face and two small bones in his hand. He looked just like a watch repairer with an extra cog wheel! What do I do with these, he asked? He did not know that among the large primates, only humans have no separate os centrale in the wrist!

Those early research interests, broadened to include clinical aspects, unwittingly pre-prepared me for participation, years later, in many research ideas and directions completely different from the original anatomical research in which I assumed I would always be involved.

A First Bone Example: Human Osteoporosis

Thus, years later in Chicago, I came to be interested in how the vertebral column may be adapted to movement in monkeys and apes. I studied spongy bone patterns in their spinal columns as part of a collaboration with a combined MD/PhD student, later surgeon Dr. Harry Yang.

This 'pre-prepared' me to look at human vertebral patterns and led to an interest in human osteoporosis. A colleague (Dr. David Johnston, University of Leeds, UK) gave me his radiographs of vertebral sections from a range of humans, with and without osteoporosis!

Figure 5.4 shows radiographs of sections of human vertebrae. Most of the spicules of bone inside a human vertebra are organized, on average, in a vertical and horizontal pattern. The radiograph

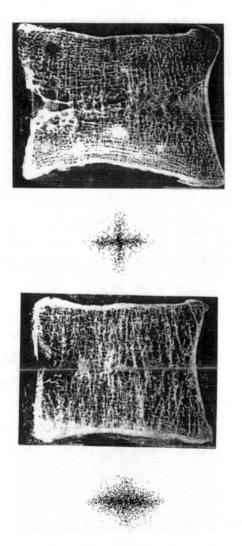

Figure 5.4: Above: a normal vertebra and its transform. Below: an osteoporotic vertebra and its transform.

above is normal: its vertical and horizontal spicules are largely equal in length. The one below shows osteoporosis. It has horizontal elements much thinner and shorter than the vertical ones.

This difference can, however, be seen and quantified much more easily by the analyses shown below each vertebra (also Figure 5.4). For normal vertebrae, these analyses (the Fourier transform) are a cross with equal arms (like a Maltese cross). This is a measure of the approximately equal sizes of the spicules of bone. In osteoporosis, where the vertical and horizontal spicule dimensions are different, the Fourier transform looks more like a rugby ball. This is the Fourier signature of osteoporosis. This difference is much more obvious in the Fourier transforms than in the original radiographs.

And it is quantifiable!

These studies, as documented more fully in another chapter, led me to understand more about how osteoporosis affects bones. It implied that it might be possible to make the diagnosis earlier than is commonly achieved, thus allowing for the possibility of lifestyle advice before the condition was serious enough to require treatment.

Of course, sadly, this information could not be used for these patients; the radiographs were obtained from the sections of road accident victims (taken with permission at postmortems).

But the same thing could be done on radiographs of bones from the living. This research all came about from the clinics. More of this story later!

More on Bones: Hearing Loss and Ear Ossicles

An ear, nose and throat surgeon, Mr. Francis Lannigan, came to Dr. (as he was then) Paul O'Higgins and me to understand more about the incus bone, one of the small bones in the ear. His surgical problem was replacing a partially resorbed incus to return hearing to a deaf patient. His question was:

"Why did the incus resorb in the first place?"

This question, from the clinic, led us to try and understand how, mechanically, the incus bone might work. The three of us started a research collaboration combining the anatomy of the ear bones, functions of bone/joint systems, and understanding of stress and strain mechanics.

First, we carried out a thought experiment to work out what was happening at the joint between the incus and the stapes. We suspected that it had something to do with the stresses close to the joint in two positions: when the incus tapped against the stapes, and when it was distracted from the stapes (Figure 5.5).

On this basis, we could 'guess' the stresses in the shaft of the incus in total, as in Figure 5.6. This guess implies that there are some parts of the bone where there are tensile stresses at all times! But this is not what bone is supposed to do. There may well be alterations between compression and tension when a bone is bent one way and then another. But tension all the time, in a compression bearing material like bone, is counterintuitive!

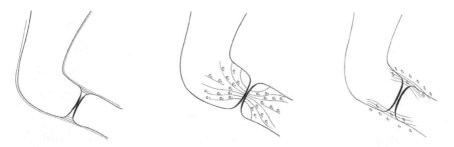

Figure 5.5: Left: joint between incus and stapes. Center: compressive stresses during the 'tap' phase of movement. Right: tensile stresses during the 'anti-tap' phase of movement.

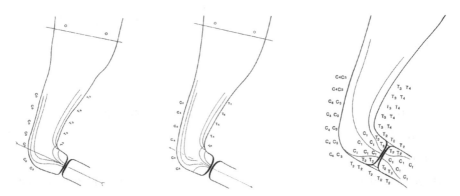

Figure 5.6:   Left: stresses in shaft and head of the incus in 'tap'. Center: in 'anti-tap'. Right: summation of stresses in both positions. C's are compressive stresses, T's are tensile stresses. The 'T's' are summed around the head and internal curve of the incus shaft!

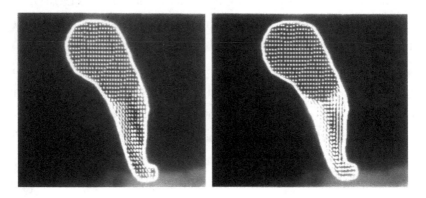

Figure 5.7:   Both pictures show tap and anti-tap, with red indicating tensile stresses. In other words, tension exists around the head in both phases of the movement.

At this point we decided that our simple thought experiment should be followed up. But we were still not yet ready to invest in a complex experiment. So, we next decided on a 'quick and dirty' but nonetheless real experiment to see what the strains might look like.

This led us to do a full-blown finite element analysis of the situation (Figure 5.7), which confirmed that some of the regions of the incus were under tension (the T's in both phases of the

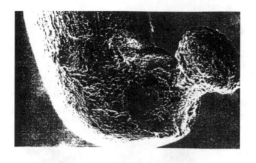

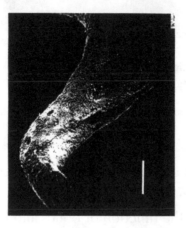

Figure 5.8: Actual bone loss around the head of the incus and on the inside of the shaft of the incus.

movement). If — and this was our hypothesis — bone was removed when under tension, we could expect bone to be removed all around the head of the incus and part-way up the concave aspect of the shaft.

Figure 5.8 shows actual loss of bone in exactly those locations in the incus.

The logic of our study is interesting and perhaps useful. First, a thought experiment; second, a simple but real experiment; third, a full-blown complex experiment; fourth, confirmation with real data. It not only saves time but also ensures that one knows what one is doing!

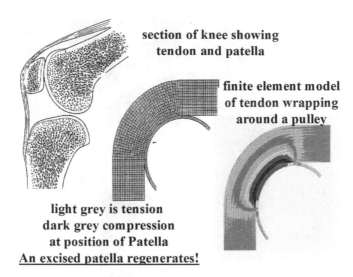

section of knee showing
tendon and patella

finite element model
of tendon wrapping
around a pulley

light grey is tension
dark grey compression
at position of Patella
An excised patella regenerates!

Figure 5.9:　Compression (dark) in a simulation of a knee (by student-then-colleague Jens Hirschberg).

These rough biomechanical studies on ear bones stemmed from earlier work examining the relationship between compression and tension in the function of bones and ligaments.

As a result, my earliest biomechanical studies came from wondering why sometimes there was bone where (I thought) there should only be tendon (e.g., the knee cap, which is a bone in a tendon, Figure 5.9).

Now for Something Completely Different: Vitamin B^{12} Deficiency

My early contacts with medical laboratory technology also pre-prepared me for totally unexpected research problems.

As I had explained above, as a young doctor, I received much help from laboratory technicians doing the many tests that we, as interns, would order for our patients. One special test involved vitamin B^{12} determinations. In those days, however, there were no direct tests as there are today. Determination of vitamin B^{12} in the patient's blood serum was through a bioassay; that is, how much vitamin B^{12} is required for *Euglena gracilis* to grow in a petri dish.

This test was not easy in those days, often taking as long as a couple of weeks. Some technicians could do it (they were said to have 'green fingers'), but others just could not, for no very obvious reason. I found out how it was done and some of the implications. When as a researcher, some of our monkeys showed paralyses, I was pre-prepared to see if it might mean deficiency of vitamin B^{12} (Figures 5.10 above and 5.11 below).

The full story is told in another chapter. The vitamin B^{12} work required me to examine pregnant rhesus monkeys, and I was quite anxious about feeling the baby through the mother's belly. I need not have worried, as I was pre-prepared. As soon as I placed my hand on my first monkey's abdomen, all the experiences of my hand on women's bellies in obstetrics came back in a rush. That

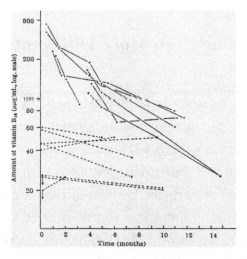

Figure 5.10: Reduction of vitamin B^{12} levels in individual monkeys over time in captivity. Newly captive animals (continuous line) are compared with long captive animals (dashed line).

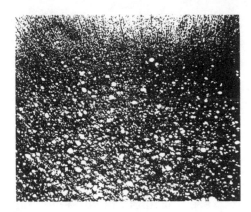

Figure 5.11: Spongy brain degeneration in a paralyzed animal due to deficiency of vitamin B^{12}.

statement is actually a cheat. A monkey's belly is so thin that anyone could feel (tongue-in-cheek) the baby's toe nails!

This all eventually led to a decade-long program of research (described in another chapter) that took me into many different aspects of vitamin B^{12} deficiency and introduced me to many new colleagues.

Next, Something Even More Different: Iodine Deficiency

My early clinical interests in bone (even as early as a fourth-year medical student) got me to look at growth problems, and this included cretinism (Figure 5.12).

Of course, cretins were no longer born in England when I was a student, because as early as the turn of that century, the cause, iodine deficiency in mothers, and the treatment, supplements for the mothers, was long known. Medical history documents that the ancient Chinese knew that seaweed (containing iodine, though they did not know that) improved some goiters (though they did not know why).

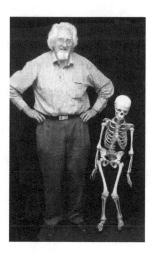

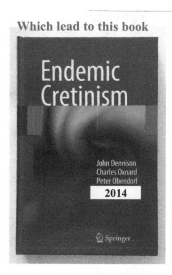

Figure 5.12:   Left: 32-year-old cretin skeleton (note the child-like breast bone). Right: the resultant book.

There should have been no 'new' cretins in my time as a UK student, but cretins could, when well looked after, live into old age. Cretinism was in the medical curriculum, and with my interests in bones, I lapped it up. Thus, when a problem related to growth deficiencies arose, I was pre-prepared to recognize cretinism. This is clearly a very important problem worldwide and is solvable with a tuppence-worth of iodine. The lifetime's work of Basil Hetzel implies that as many as two billion people are at risk of iodine deficiency, one billion may have goiters, and many more than ten million may be cretins.

Finally, Most Different of All: Forensics

Inevitably, someone whose training has included human anatomy and medicine is likely to be involved in forensics. For all Birmingham students, it started when we took forensic medicine and toxicology in the fifth year with Prof. Webster. His subject, and his lecturing style, were so exciting that his lecture room was always full to the brim. People (not all medical students; many others from around the locality would sneak in) would even be sitting on the stairs and around the dais at the front.

I have never forgotten Prof. Webster showing a slide of the body of a young woman, lying on her back in the bushes, the result of a rape-murder, with her nether regions covered with a raincoat. The raincoat, he explained, was to avoid upsetting the medical students.

Next slide please — the same picture without the raincoat. It brought down the house. I'm sure this couldn't be done today.

A little later, when a new hospital was being built in Birmingham, on the site of an old deconsecrated cemetery, I had to climb down the walls of the hole being made for the foundations. I had to certify that the little rushes of water were the digger entering old grave chambers, and not new murders.

Then there was an occasion in Birmingham when I admitted a heavily jaundiced individual into casualty (today, emergency). He looked as though he was about to die, but I had no idea what was wrong with him. So, I took about 120ccs of blood and divvied it up amongst about a dozen or more tests! He did indeed die. By good fortune (mine, not his), one of the tests showed what was wrong: he had Weil's disease, an infection by the organism, *leptospirosis ictero haemorrhagica.*

At that time, any casualty death within 4 hours became a coroner's case. I was therefore summoned to court as an expert witness to certify the cause of death. But this was not an ordinary coroner's court. This was the high court acting as a coroner's court — the reason: a matter of public safety.

The organism in Weil's disease is carried by rats and spread in their urine. The deceased was a farmer (lots of rats in farms), had been digging ditches (rats were common around ditches), was a keen ferreter (ferrets also carry the organism), *and he worked part-time in the meat market in town!* The whole case was to show that, however he got it, the meat market in town was clean. No rats there.

(What the court did not know was that I also visited the meat market in town for pig fetuses for my research. "Here, catch these," the butcher would say, slashing open the abdomen of a dead pregnant sow. As a result of these visits, however, I knew that place was overrun with rats. But I was just an expert witness [a so-called expert] about the cause of death, nothing else. You answer what you are asked, you don't volunteer.)

I remember being asked the cause of death. I started to say, "Hepatic failure, Your Honor," but I had only gotten the first syllable ("hep-") out of my mouth when there was a loud cough from the well of the court. It was my forensic medicine professor, Old Webster, catching my attention. I quickly amended my words to "liver failure, Your Honor." Use simple words, Webster had taught us.

In Chicago, we had a program that permitted students from any of the Chicago universities to take courses *for free* at any other university if that course was not available in their own institution. The courses I gave were unique to the University of Chicago. So, students from other places took my courses. I once gave a mark of 10 to a student from Northwestern University for a research paper in this course. I had never given 10 — the top mark — before.

The student was Kathy Reichs, who years later would write a series of highly successful books, television programs, and so on. I particularly remember her first book, *Death Du Jour*, the French words being because she did her forensic work in Canada! Years later we were in contact again, and she remembered that ten. When I (respectfully) asked for her news of her next production, she sent me a photograph of her grandchild!

Again, years later when I was in Los Angeles, there was a spate of deaths amongst black citizens due to police tactics for subduing them. The police were using two methods. One was called the carotid hold, consisting of a bent elbow being employed around the neck to compress the carotid artery. The other was called the arm-bar hold, where the forearm was pressed horizontally across the trachea (reminiscent of the recent US case).

There were a number of fatalities, which also, of course, caused great anger in the community. Accordingly, the then-Chief of Police (named Bradley, as I remember it) was interviewed by the press.

"Why were so many black people dying?"

was the question.

"Oh," he said,

"it's the anatomy of the neck. *Blacks* don't have necks like *normal* people." The words *blacks* and *normal* certainly hit a nerve!

Immediately the press looked for an anatomist who might know about the anatomy of the neck. Who then but me — the only medically qualified anatomist around. I was so worried. I was interviewed in our beautiful garden in Pasadena for television, and they filmed me answering questions for about 40 minutes. But I knew that they would only show about two minutes on telly. Which two minutes would they show? I need not have worried; they were on my side.

Early in my time in Western Australia, I was involved with Len Friedman in examining some burnt bone fragments for the police. They had been found in the bush. The question was: were these the remnants of a legitimate indigenous cremation, or the result of a murder?

The pieces were very small — as though they had been smashed. There were only two pieces we could identify with certainty: both the lower ends of the radius. We knew this because of the bony tubercle (Lister's tubercle) on the radius around which loops a tendon going to the thumb. There was a problem, however: the one fragment was almost twice the size of the other! And the modes of burning seemed to have been different for each, possibly at different temperatures. Were these reflecting more than one cremation attempt, more than one individual involved, or possibly even at more than one time? Well, the police didn't seem to want to know. So, this never went anywhere!

Very late in my career, my knowledge of bone and bones has involved me rather more fully with forensic medicine (again as detailed elsewhere). As a result, I have had the pleasure of a whole series of new investigations with forensic colleagues (especially the forensic anthropologist Dr. Daniel Franklin; first my research fellow, then my collaborator, then my mentor, and now my professor. So, do roles become reversed). Dan wanted to know: how can one tell from bones whether the specimen is animal or human, or male or female (Figure 5.13), or even the age at death or its possible ethnicity?

All this brought back to me my remembrance of the time when I was a law school dropout (Chapter 2).

The Importance of the Triad Idea

I have enjoyed all these, and many other, clinically related investigations — so different from my initial research interests and involving so many new disciplines, so many new technologies, and so many new students and colleagues.

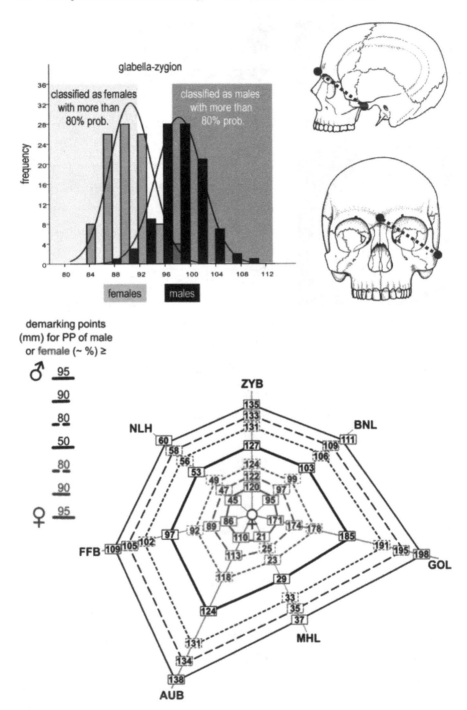

Figure 5.13:   classifying sex in skulls with a single measurement. The bell-shaped curves indicate what we all know: that there is much overlap between the sexes. The seven-dimensional results showing much better sexing by using many measurements.

I would not have done any of this had I been *only* a teacher, *only* a researcher, or even *only* a practicing physician alone. It has, further, moved the well-known teaching/research nexus into a teaching/research/practice triad!

It required:

an unusual medico-scientific background,
accidental introductions to totally new technologies and disciplines,
many collaborations with undergraduates, graduates and research fellows, and
much networking with professionals, doctors, technicians and other scientists.

They have been so important to my value to the students, and my enjoyment of the work.

Part 3
Research Wrinkles
Chapters 6–12

A standard view of research is that it is a surefooted, deliberate, step by step process for finding things out and getting things done. It is as though researchers make observations, do experiments, churn out hard cold facts, patiently piecing together a giant jig-saw puzzle. Scientists are confirming big ideas, answering big questions, recording big advances, all the themes of popular science programmes.

Unfortunately, this leads to the idea that research is the accumulation of facts and the confirmation of ideas. **And we, ourselves, reinforce it if we teach by emphasizing regurgitating facts and accepting ideas!**

These are indeed a part of research, but by no means the whole story. They do not show the day-to-day, nitty gritty, in the office, at the clinic, by the computer, on the bench, parts of research. They do not show what gets us into the lab early and what keeps us there late. They certainly do not show that our real aim is to kill ideas, sometimes by making observations, sometimes by doing experiments, sometimes just by thinking. Old ideas die; new ideas are born. And new ideas may not simply be slight embellishments of the old. They sometimes involve totally new insights. And they are to be tested in their turn! The entire thing is a roundabout of thought and action, thought and action.

This may have been best put by Donald Rumsfeld, US Department of Defense.

"There are known knowns. These are things that we know we know."
"There are known unknowns. These are things that we know we don't know."
"And there are unknown unknowns. These are things we don't know we don't know."

In other words, research happens in many ways. It is more hit and miss than you would imagine. There is much stumbling and groping. My own researches exemplify it in spades! Perhaps we ought to tell students more often what really happens in research most of the time.

Chapter 6: "Just Sheer Dumb Luck" (Professor McGonagall, Hogwarts)

Chapter 7: Borrowed, Gifted, Shared, Even Invented (But Not Stolen!)

Chapter 8: Three Heresies and Thrice a Heretic!

Chapter 9: Guessing Human Pasts, 'Guestimating' Human Futures

Chapter 10: Gold Standards, Accepted Wisdoms, Best Practices: Are they Crippling Straitjackets?

Chapter 11: 'O-metrics': Finding What is Hidden!

Chapter 12: International Links: Especially China!

6 "Just Sheer Dumb Luck" (Professor Mcgonagall, Hogwarts)

One day a fellow graduate student in psychology (Malcolm Roberts, now Emeritus Professor Roberts) came to me with a peculiar request. Would I, as a young physician, look after his monkeys medically? He had just imported a dozen green monkeys for psychological research. This was in a time when it was allowed.

What more natural, in those days, than that I should help — no skin off my nose, no boundary disputes with vets, no payment required!

These poor creatures — kept for weeks in holding facilities in Africa after capture, travelling cooped up in small crates, held on arrival at Shamrock Farms on the south coast of England awaiting transport to Birmingham — were in a terrible condition. Some had died in transit. The rest had diarrhea and vomiting, were coughing and sneezing, and were thin, scruffy and listless. I was sure they had ectoparasites; I guessed they had enteroparasites too. Worst of all, they could not speak and tell me what was wrong. **It was like paediatrics all over again!**

> *When I did paediatrics I thought that if a small child looked well, it was probably ill, and if it looked ill, it was going to die.*

This applies even more to a small monkey! I agreed to treat them.

I gave sulphonamides for the gut infections, penicillin for the lung infections, and vitamins because they looked as though they needed them (all of which I obtained gratis, from the hospital dispensary; no 'user pays' in those days!), together with good food. I was careful not to fall into the trap of treating their parasites immediately; that was to wait until they were strong enough to take those powerful drugs. This was not particularly clever, just blockbuster treatment with precious little diagnosis. They got better and Malcolm was delighted.

The Value of Luck, Error, Failure, and Eating our Words!

"An ingenious conjecture greatly shortens the road."
Gottfried Wilhelm Leibnitz, 1646–1716.

"Truth comes out of error more readily than out of confusion."
Francis Bacon, 1620.

"When all else fails, read the 'destructions'!"
(My wife's words!)

Now it happened that I had included folic acid as one of the vitamins in the diet of these monkeys. This instantly tells you that I did not know much about monkeys or diets. Eating mainly plant materials as they do, the one thing they would not be short of was folic acid!

Soon after, I was called to see a rhesus monkey that had been in our colony for a long time. It had become paralyzed in its hind legs and tail.

"I'm afraid nothing can be done,"
said I, making the 'snap' diagnosis of 'cage paralysis'! I knew this occasionally occurred in monkeys.

Then the technician who called me admitted, *very bravely*:

"You know you ordered folic acid for the new green monkeys. By mistake I gave folic acid to this rhesus monkey."

Of course, that reminded me of humans where giving folic acid to a patient with pernicious anaemia, a vitamin B^{12} deficiency problem, can precipitate a paralysis called sub-acute combined degeneration of the cord (I was the sort of medical student who read all the footnotes!). The excess folic acid channels what little B^{12} there is toward the blood-forming system, leaving the nervous system deficient.

"Perhaps the monkey is deficient in vitamin B^{12}?"

I mused.

"Let's give it a shot".

The animal got a bit better. Of course, having given it B^{12}, I could not test for deficiency.

O' foolish physician! We were no wiser.

Shortly after, another monkey 'spontaneously' showed 'cage paralysis'. This time I did the right thing: I checked the vitamin B^{12} levels first. The result: 25 picograms/ml (the normal human level is 200–600). The monkey was clearly deficient! *Or was it? Perhaps monkeys are different?* So, I started a new research project on the weekends.

Weekends were an especial time for research in Zuckerman's Department. After all, he was busy in Whitehall for much of the normal week (see another chapter), so weekends were all that he had. If you wanted him to know you were working, you worked on the weekends!

I did not know the normal values for monkeys, so I tested a further dozen of our 'normal' monkeys. Surprise: all had levels below 100. Did this mean that all our monkeys were deficient? Or was this normal, and monkeys are different from humans? Was the improvement of the treated animal a red herring? So, I started reading more about vitamin B^{12}.

Humans and pigs have levels of 200 to 600, sheep and cows in the 1,000s, rabbits in the 40,000s. Nothing seems to have levels below 150 except for certain cases, such as people with untreated pernicious anaemia and its rare complication of subacute combined degeneration of the spinal cord, people with infestation with the fish tapeworm (that selectively absorbs the B^{12} that should go to the host), people with surgically created blind pockets or loops in the gut, people with certain complications of pregnancy, people who are true vegans(!), AND our rhesus monkeys! Yet, of course, I still could not be certain.

I therefore visited Shamrock Farms on the South Coast of England where, in those days, imported monkeys arrived in the United Kingdom. This clinched the matter. Blood from some 20 recently arrived rhesus monkeys showed that they were similar to normal humans. Thus, *almost all* our monkeys (eventually several hundred were tested) were deficient, paralyzed or not!

Many questions arose from these findings. What was the cause of the deficiency? How did it develop? What happened upon treatment of deficient animals? What about the two animals with cage paralysis? What was the picture in other monkey species? What were the implications for the many different scientific investigations carried out on these monkeys over the years? Did this problem also exist in other research monkey colonies, and in zoos? Were there implications for the field situation? Were there implications for evolution?

These were among the plethora of questions I tried to answer in the next two decades.

The Full Vitamin B¹² Story

But I needed to know more about vitamin B^{12} itself. My newly acquired medical knowledge was not good enough. I was here aided by Lester Smith, a Glaxo Laboratories biochemist (a colleague of Nobel Prize winner Dorothy Hodgkin, who worked out the molecular structure of vitamin B^{12}).

I knew so little that Lester Smith even had to tell me that vitamin B^{12} is not an ordinary 'B' vitamin. It is involved in many fundamental biochemical reactions in a wide array of living things. Most relate to microorganisms in soil, dirt, garbage, feces and sewage sludge.

"Half the secret of disease resistance is cleanliness; the other half is dirtiness!"

Why Do We Need Vitamin B¹² and How Do We Get It?

There are at least two functions of vitamin B^{12} in humans. One is support of cell division for growth, the other is support for white nerve fiber function for the passage of impulses.

So, where do the different mammals get their vitamin B^{12}? Carnivores, omnivores, and your average humans get B^{12} from eating animal foods. As there is no B^{12} in plants, herbivores get their B^{12} in other ways. In cows and sheep, for example, B^{12} is first produced in the stomach by microorganisms, and then absorbed beyond in the small intestine. Guinea pigs get B^{12} by eating their own soft fecal pellets at night, thus returning vitamin B^{12} produced by microorganisms in the colon to the small intestine via the mouth! Rabbits, by reverse peristalsis, return vitamin from the very large blind appendix back up to the small intestine.

The nutritional requirements of B^{12}, whatever the animal and whatever the blood levels, are actually very small. As a result, a dietary lack takes years to produce a blood deficiency.

But dietary lacks do tend to occur in poorly fed residents in nursing homes or other institutions (therefore vitamin B^{12} deficiency is often found in the aged). They also tend occur in true vegetarians, including their fetuses and babies! It does not occur in those less strict vegetarians who, while eschewing meat, still take animal products like milk, eggs and fish (all contain the vitamin).

The deficiency may also occur in humans in various medical conditions. These include pernicious anaemia (due to auto-immune stomach damage), infection with the B^{12} absorbing fish tapeworm (especially common in Scandinavia and Japan) in raw fish eaters, as a complication of various surgical procedures on the gut, as a side effect of older treatments for peptic ulcers (perhaps from eliminating the source of stomach factors also necessary for absorption of vitamin B^{12}), after removal of the small intestine (as in the older treatments of Krohn's disease), and after the surgical creation of bowel cul-de-sacs!

Deficiency can be produced in coprophagic (feces-eating) animals by heroic measures such as preventing coprophagy with body splints that stop them from getting the mouth to the anus at night, or by chemically stressing them (e.g., giving thyroid hormone) to increase B^{12} requirements.

My Initial Results

I would take blood on Fridays. In the beginning, samples were analyzed (in Dr. Marshall Chalmers' laboratory in the Queen Elizabeth Hospital, Birmingham; he was willing to help a young physician *gratis*); results were available two weeks later.

So, Monday morning coffee time two weeks later was when I reported the findings to my fellow research students. There was usually news to report and, as it also happened, *old errors to recant!*

In our monkey colony, the vitamin levels in the monkeys on entry quickly reduced, at a logarithmic rate (Figure 6.1), to the same levels as in seriously deficient humans.

This also occurred in many other primates (most from the London Zoological Society). The species differences started to confirm the cause of the deficiency. Thus, pottos, lorises, bush babies and lemurs had good blood levels however long captive, because they are largely insectivorous and will not live unless given

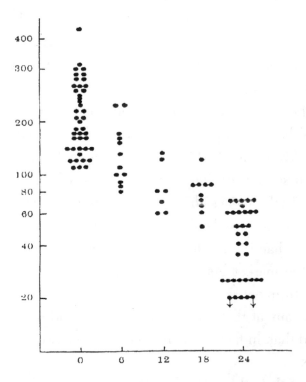

Figure 6.1: Amount of Vitamin B^{12} on the Y (vertical) axis (note the logarithmic scale on this axis) in rhesus monkeys with time in months since arrival, on the X (horizontal) axis.

animal foods. The few leaf-eating monkeys had high levels of the vitamin and, of course, they have sacculated stomachs operating somewhat like in cows and sheep as previously described.

But most monkeys and apes, when recently captive, had levels like normal humans. Those captive for more than 2 years were like our long-captive rhesus monkeys.

There were several interesting individual exceptions. First, a fall in levels with time in captivity did not occur in our green monkeys; but these were the ones I had given vitamin B^{12} and fed good food on entry. Second, a reduction did not occur in one of the London gibbons. It turned out that this animal received one ounce of meat daily from its keeper. Third, two baboons from the London Zoo were not deficient. They were kept outside for much of the year and, in addition to plant foods provided by the keepers, also ate whatever they could find outside: insects, birds and birds' eggs, small rodents, and discarded food from zoo visitors. Finally, one chimpanzee had very high levels every time its blood was examined. But Desmond Morris (then at the London Zoo) told me that this animal had developed fecal pica (the habit of eating its own feces). *All this implied that it must be a simple dietary deficiency?*

Of course, this was long before the days of commercial monkey chows. In those days, the staff of a university research monkey colony (thinking, mistakenly, that a monkey is an animal with a banana in its hand) often found it cheaper to buy fruit late in the day from the market. As a result, at that time, our animals were vegetarian from entry.

And again, at that time in the 1950s, it had not been clearly recognized that, in fact, many monkeys normally eat some animal food items.

It was only in the 1960s that Jane Goodall's findings of termite 'fishing' by chimpanzees became well known. The 1930s sighting of this by Fred Merfield, Colonel Powell-Cotton's 'shooter', had been overlooked. So, too, was a Liberian postage stamp (1906) showing a chimpanzee 'fishing', which came from a drawing by Gustav Mutzell (1887) of a chimpanzee 'fishing' in Dresden Zoo (Figure 6.2).

Of course, this deficiency should not occur today because captive animals are fed monkey chows. Chows contain offal that, being an animal product, is loaded with vitamin B^{12}. In fact, within 6 weeks of my second paper in *Nature*, the monkey chow company

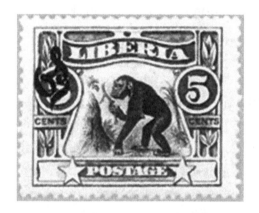

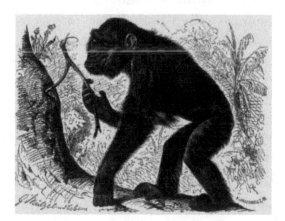

Figure 6.2: Liberian postage stamp (1906) showing chimpanzee 'fishing', and the drawing by Gustav Mutzell (1887) on which it looks as though it was based!

changed the label on their product to read 'vitamin B^{12} added'! They did not know that this was unnecessary because of the offal content of their chows. I did not know that this was a patentable idea; otherwise I might now be royalty rich!

However, though we had identified a dietary deficiency, there were still many questions.

Hidden B^{12} Deficiency I: Sex, Pregnancy and Babies

Studies of reproduction (by Zuckerman, Krohn, Eckstein, Mandl and many others in Birmingham) were the main reasons for the existence of the Birmingham monkey colony.

Was vitamin B^{12} relevant to reproduction? Among the monkeys on entry, the pregnant or puerperal ones already had reduced vitamin B^{12} levels. Is it possible that the levels in field diets may be marginal enough (seasonal changes for example) that the advent of pregnancy (with the fetus parasitizing the mother for the vitamin) produces a deficiency in the mother? This would be temporary; eating the placenta, for example, would immediately replenish the mother's supply. Further, though injecting B^{12} (as therapy) in non-pregnant animals raised their levels, in pregnant animals it did not raise the mothers' levels, but it did raise the levels in their fetuses, presumably being passed on through.

But there was more. Fertility, in our colony, had always been low. We never had as many babies as we should have! There are many likely reasons (environmental, physical, social and psychological) for this. But our monkeys' reproductive cycles were irregular. Old records showed that the cycles were not simply irregular; they were 'regularly irregular', seemingly due to single, double or, even on occasion, triple missed cycles. Could it be that pregnancies occurred but failed early with resorption of embryos and a return to cycling?

All this made it prudent to look further. It was already known in both normal humans and cattle that vitamin B^{12} content was high in semen and blastocysts, and that reduced vitamin B^{12} in the semen and blastocyst fluid was associated with reduced fertility. It was known that B^{12} had to be added to bull semen used for artificial insemination in cattle.

Moreover, as a young clinician, I was aware that women with pernicious anaemia (usually in early middle age) should be 'warned' that they should, in the language of those days, 'take precautions' if they did not wish to become pregnant soon after B^{12} treatment!

The overall upshot of these studies was the idea that the deficiency was associated with problems in reproduction, but the evidence at the time was not sufficient to be sure.

Hidden B^{12} Deficiency II: Skin, Blood and Bones

Doctors should always look at patients' faces and in their mouths. Some monkeys had fissures at the corners of the mouth (angular cheilosis), smooth tongues (glossitis), and white patches on gums (stomatitis), all confirmed for me by a dental colleague, Dr. Margaret Rose.

It later turned out that such features were not only present in the mouth, but also in the epithelium of the rest of the gut. They may also have been present elsewhere, for example, the cervix, vagina and uterus. But I didn't know because I did not then think of examining those sites! Such changes are due to interference with cell growth.

Thus, the blood, continually proliferating, shows changes. In humans, the commonest manifestation in blood is pernicious anaemia. Our animals did not have this. More detailed blood studies of the deficient animals were all statistically similar to recently captive monkeys and normal humans. In other words, anaemia like that of pernicious anaemia in humans (enlarged red cells) seems not to occur in rhesus monkeys.

> *Of course, I published this. Almost immediately*
> *I had to eat my words.*

It was not that the original observations were wrong. It was rather that, later, when we compared each animal with itself before and after treatment, we found that indeed there were significant changes. The red blood cells were indeed larger after treatment, but the degree was so small that we could only show it by comparing the same animal before and after (through collaboration with another clinical colleague, Dr. Eric Spicer).

> *Of course, this meant publishing another paper.*

Given these problems in skin and blood, I could logically expect that there would also be interference in growth generally. It was well known that giving vitamin B^{12} (e.g., to farm animals) increased their size, so deficiency reduces growth. It was not, however, such published information that led me to look at growth.

It was rather, once more, a series of *accidental observations* made during attempts to discover the minimum dose of vitamin B^{12} needed to maintain blood levels.

I had given small doses of the vitamin to three infants on a regular basis over some months while monitoring vitamin levels. The doses given were so small that after an initial surge in blood levels of the vitamin in the days following each injection, the levels fell back. I did it three times in each infant, and then plotted changes in weight with age. Weights surged shortly following injection and then, shortly after that, fell back. Over three cycles, this gave a saw-toothed curve. It seems reasonable that the B^{12} injections caused surges in growth.

Of course, I published this. Again, I had to eat my words.

This was because I found that three other rhesus babies not given the vitamin, a very small control group of course, had been weighed at the same time. To my chagrin, they showed precisely the same saw-toothed curve of weight on age. In other words, the original finding was little more than an accident — the samples were too small, many other secular factors in the colony could have been involved, and it may not have been true anyway!

Therefore, with another colleague, Dr. Roger Flinn, we did a properly controlled study of growth. The results were startling. In both sexes, growth, after regularly giving the vitamin, was so increased that we thought that we might have to order bigger cages! The changes were clearly large enough to be important in the rearing of monkeys in captivity.

Yet another paper was required!

Note: find your mistakes before someone else does!

Hidden B^{12} Deficiency III: Nerves, Spinal Cord and Brain

By far the most interesting sign of deficiency in captive monkeys was damage to the nervous system (quite rare in humans).

In human cases of reduced vitamin B^{12} levels, the blood problems predominate. But a small number of humans may show subacute combined degeneration of the (spinal) cord. This complication, when it occurs, is a dire emergency. Patients complain of pins and needles in the feet, have changed leg reflexes, and have weak or even paralyzed legs. This worsens over just days and becomes permanent unless treated with vitamin B^{12}.

Our deficient monkeys were different. Following the initial diagnosis of 'cage paralysis' in the two animals that started all this, we discovered, over a two-year period, that many (more than forty) developed neurological symptoms.

The symptoms were consistent. The animals, could they speak, might have complained of pins and needles in their feet (and tails). They usually sat with their feet turned in so that the soles did not touch the cage floor. Some had self-inflicted wounds on their feet and tails. Both of these are possibly evidence of paraesthesiae.

The worst cases could only drag themselves around the cages seemingly from partial leg paralyses. In the less-affected animals, mobility was impaired, resulting in clumsy climbing with apparent difficulty. Sometimes the limbs showed a tremor. Sometimes they had difficulty handling a small object, such as a nut; was this a loss of manual dexterity, evidence of a visual problem, or both?

Neurological signs in monkeys are not easy to obtain, though they are a bit easier if the monkeys are paralyzed. Yet the signs there were. Touching the feet caused distress. Their legs seemed weak. There were changed nerve reflexes, initially exaggerated but later reduced.

Of course, the paralyzed animals were the first I examined postmortem. When I first removed a spinal cord and brain, it took me 57 minutes. Eventually I could do it in 7 minutes! The initial histology was done by the neuropathologist, Professor Walter Smith, but most of the later histology was by our joint doctoral student, Dr. Ildemaro Torres Nŭnez (professor of anatomy in his own country, Venezuela).

We first looked at leg nerves (Figure 6.3). The axons had lost their insulating cover (demyelination) and this was worst further down the leg. We therefore thought that the deficiency affected

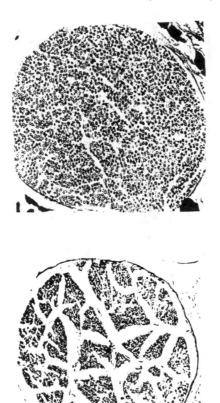

Figure 6.3: Sections of leg nerves stained for nerve fibers in a recently captive animal (above), and in a long-stay monkey (below).

the nerve cell body so that it could not support such a long length of axon. The nerve fibers were dying back to a length that could be supported by the cell body.

We published this finding (and it is indeed correct).

Yet again, however, we had to eat our words!

This was because we had examined the worst-affected cases first, a natural thing to do. It was this that suggested a die-back phenomenon, the Wallerian degeneration.

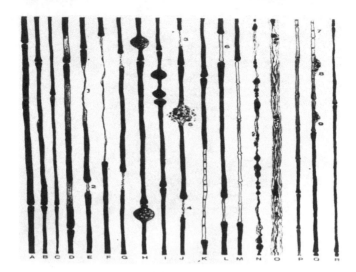

Figure 6.4:   A series of teased nerve fibers. Only the fiber on the left is normal. All the rest show demyelination of various degrees.

However, looking later at less affected animals showed that this die-back was secondary to demyelination due to supporting (Schwann) cell damage. Ildemaro, teasing individual nerve fibers (something I had done earlier in my dissection of a shrew!), showed the lesions to be segmental (Figure 6.4).

All this required another paper!

We also examined the deficient but non-paralyzed animals. To our utter surprise, every one showed damage to nerves of the lower limbs and spinal cord, but of less degree (Figure 6.5). And we eventually carried out a wide-ranging survey of the whole nervous system.

There were similar problems in the nerve cells in the retina, in the optic nerves, in the white matter of the cerebral cortex (Figure 6.6), and passing to the optic area of the occipital lobe of the brain.

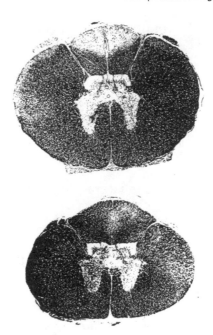

Figure 6.5: Upper frame: the badly damaged spinal cord (white parts) of a paralyzed monkey. Lower frame: the slightly damaged spinal cord (the lessened white parts) of a monkey without paralysis.

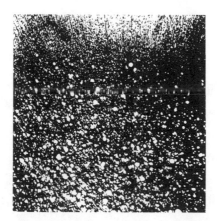

Figure 6.6: Similar spongy-like degeneration in the cerebral cortex.

This latter work stemmed from the doctoral thesis of yet another collaborator, ophthalmologist Dr. Valerie Hinds.

The incidence of nervous system lesions in these vitamin B_{12}-deficient animals was virtually 100%. Yet, of all these animals, not a single one had the full-blown large cell anaemia of humans. The relationship between lesions of blood and brain was thus opposite to humans.

All this work led to some lateral thinking: a *sine qua non* for research!

The Importance of Lateral Thinking

Lateral Thinking: Evolutionary Ideas

What did this difference between monkeys and humans mean? In most monkeys in the field, the primary diets are a variety of plant foods. It is only occasional that animal products are obtained, and when they are, they are often shared very unequally. A dominant male, a favorite consort and her baby, may get the lion's share, while most of the others get scraps or nothing. As a result, vitamin B_{12} levels are likely marginal in most animals, so many fairly quickly become deficient when on a vegetarian diet in captivity.

Further, folic acid availability must also be considered because, in the field, the food is primarily plants, so folic acid will be present in abundance. The cell growth systems (e.g., blood, bone, skin) require both vitamin B_{12} and folic acid. The brain needs vitamin B_{12} alone. Thus, in the presence of excess folic acid, if there is only a little vitamin B_{12}, it is channeled toward growth. As a result, the nervous system may be starved.

Perhaps, in the field, such animals are on the verge of B_{12} deficiency coupled with folic acid excess most of the time. This may not matter much because changes in conditions (eating a small amount of animal food occasionally, eating the placenta, and even eating earth, and earth-contaminated roots and tubers) can restore reduced values of B^{12}. In contrast, humans are mostly omnivorous, and have been for millions of years.

If we look at fossils, we see information about diet. Thus, though the members of the genus *Australopithecus* were likely mainly vegetarian (see their large fibrous plant-crushing teeth), members of the genus *Homo* (with much smaller and fewer teeth) were presumably not. The taking of animal foods may have started with scavenging by groups of pre-humans long before hunting. As a result, pre-humans may have had much larger dietary amounts of vitamin B^{12} than pre-apes or australopithecines. Hence, they may have had larger stores of the vitamin. Certainly, a vegetarian diet takes a long time to produce a deficiency in modern humans.

However, this could have further important implications. The brains of modern apes and australopithecines are at the upper end of a trend toward increasing brain size in nonhuman primates. Humans, however, are enormously further evolved in this direction than either of these.

Is it possible that the precarious vitamin B^{12} status of apes may be one factor (out of many) limiting the size and complexity of their brains? And if this is true for today's apes, it may have also been true for other largely vegetarian fossil creatures (like *Paranthropus* and *Australopithecus*). It may well have been the unique (among primates) onset of an omnivorous diet at some point in pre-human lineages that supplied the vitamin B^{12} conditions that removed this constraint. This (allied with other factors, see other chapters) may have allowed one or more 'cerebral rubicons' to be crossed in pre-humans.

Could this new metabolic background have been at least one of the factors that allowed changes in the brain involving not only increased size, but also increased complexity, in humans?

Is it possible that such a dietary limitation was one among probably many factors that prevented human-like increases in size and complexity in apes and australopithecines?

Lateral Thinking Again: Medical Possibilities

There is also a medical story that stems from these studies. The beginning of the nervous system in the very early embryo is a gutter — the neural groove — on the back. This gutter then moves under the skin to become a tube, the neural tube. This tube eventually becomes the spinal cord and brain. When folic acid is deficient, this tube remains partially open and gives rise to a severe malformation, spina bifida (a neural tube defect). It is unlikely that this could occur in monkeys; their high dietary intakes of folic acid ought to prevent it. In human mothers, however, it may occur, but supplementation of the mothers' diets with folic acid prevents it.

This folic acid/spina bifida/neural tube defect link was noted in the late 1990s by Professor Fiona Stanley's group (then the Research Institute for Child Health, Western Australia). As a result, supplementation with folic acid has long been a health policy in Western Australia, and now, everywhere! Reducing the incidence of such defects in babies has been successful.

However, consider the following scenario. Sixty years ago (the 1960s), I was studying vitamin B^{12} in monkeys. I was particularly working with pregnant monkeys, and with their fetuses and babies. I was measuring the transplacental passage of vitamin B^{12}. I was trying to assay folic acid to look at relationships with B^{12}. I was involved in the pathology of the brain.

Question: why did I not discover that spina bifida could be prevented with folic acid?

Why not indeed?

Of course, it is possible that I might not have had the perspicacity to see the problem.

But if I had not, perhaps one of my colleagues or students might.

One cannot say. But we did not make the discovery.

But the real reason is because the work stopped. Why?

First, there was the matter of cost. The cost of a rhesus monkey went from £10.00 each in the UK to the thousands (in dollars) in the USA. The cost of food went from buying it oneself in the market at the end of the day to paying for a very expensive central feeding system. The cost of shelter increased from keeping them in an inexpensive, nonprofit-making, departmental colony to keeping them in an expensive central animal holding facility that (under the then new ETOB policies — 'each tub on its own bottom') had to recover all costs and, indeed, make a profit. The cost of medical treatment by a young physician (me) at no charge changed to the cost of care by extremely expensive veterinarians. The costs of tests went from courtesy service by medical laboratory colleagues to high costs in a veterinary pathology unit. Even the costs of drugs went from gifted drugs from our pharmacy to officially ordered and paid-for drugs. 'Collegial courtesy' gave way to the 'bottom line' and 'user pays'.

Second, the work might well have been carried on by the Agricultural Research Council (ARC), UK (the source of some of my original research funds). Indeed, they tried to do this. They spent a lot of money attempting to create the vitamin deficiency in their animals over a three-year period. Unfortunately, I had left the UK for the USA. The ARC was trying to do it with baboons (kept outdoors), not rhesus monkeys (inside). I may have been, at that time, perhaps the only person in the world who knew that this could not be done because of animal foods obtained in the outdoors situation.

As a result, the ARC follow-up with baboons was abandoned.

Third, my own further participation was abandoned because of the increasing activities of the animal rights lobby. One effect of the 'gentle' wing of that lobby was important: the improvement of conditions under which the animals were kept. Improvements were certainly needed. However, improvements came with increased bureaucracy, long delays and high costs. They eventually stopped most work on primates.

Good ideas may have bad effects.

Fourth, a far more serious effect stemmed from the 'violent' wing of animal rights groups. It simply became too dangerous to do this kind of work. The Wisconsin Animal Facility (this was just up the road from the University of Chicago where I was at the time) was bombed by protesters. Experimental animals were 'freed' into the Wisconsin winter. Poor things! Five years' worth of data for a doctoral thesis were destroyed. I seem to remember that someone was killed. Other similar facilities were similarly treated. This is still happening. I have colleagues who are incommunicado, even into retirement, due to threats from such groups.

This is not a grumble against animal rights. Improvements in animal handling, the ethics of experimentation, the running of facilities, and protections of both animals and staff are necessary. But because of how it occurred, our work was forced to stop in the 1970s.

Forty years of damaged babies might have been avoided! A lot of families might have been spared anguish with normal babies born instead!

Lateral Thinking a Third Time: An Even Broader Possibility

A final thought intrudes. Zuckerman had set up the animal colony to tackle a range of applied problems of breeding, hormones, fertility, contraception and so on, all of great significance to humanity. Many of these studies on what were thought to be normals, have never been reexamined in the light of these findings! Indeed, I once heard it said that it did not matter: *"After all, a monkey is just a walking womb!"*

Was Professor McGonagall Right?

Was Professor McGonagall right in describing Harry Potter's actions as "just sheer dumb luck?" How much of this is descriptive of research?

7 Borrowed, Gifted, Shared, Even Invented (But Not Stolen!)

Chapter

My first research area, human anatomy, may be the oldest of the sciences. It was mostly investigated with scalpels and forceps. These instruments, and the naked eye, showed what could be seen beneath the skin. Quite early on, the eye was extended by the hand lens and then the microscope.

By my time, these methods were greatly augmented. Sometimes these came from anatomists themselves, but very largely they were borrowed from outside anatomy. The story is often told about how the technique of percussing the chest was borrowed from percussing a barrel to estimate the level of the wine. X-rays, for imaging anatomy, stemmed from physics and radioactivity.

And just as methods could be borrowed, so too, could ideas. Borrowing ideas (one might call it stealing, perhaps) is a research method that I have used many times. Attending disciplinary meetings other than one's own, discussing problems with colleagues in unrelated subjects, looking for parallels (e.g., parallels between structures of oil-bearing rocks and marrow-bearing bones), and many other examples of borrowing, have been grist to my mill.

Pictures of Anatomies

Most of the modern improvements in anatomy involved pictures. The electron microscope and its various guises, such as the scanning electron microscope, the tunnelling electron microscope, and even more recent 'microscopes' including fluorescent, confocal, and x-ray microscopes, all came along.

To these have now been added three-dimensional imaging (electronic and computational), three-dimensional printing (objects), video imaging (moving), and functional imaging (showing functions of imaged structures).

None of these were available when I was a student. They take our understanding from the whole body through organs, tissues and cells, to intracellular structures, to macromolecules, ions even atoms and subatomic particles, and to changes in all of these with function, and over time.

They have been a fantastic set of changes during my lifetime. One might wonder why I did not go in these directions. Certainly, many of my students did.

But when I was a medical student, I rather quickly found that the microscope did not suit me. I just seemed not to be able to see clearly what other students saw immediately.

I only passed the histology examination by examining the microscope slides with a hand lens (or the microscope eye-piece), a technique that, for most purposes (in those days), could tell me what I was seeing. It was only many years later, when I came to develop longer and longer arms (I mean of course the onset of presbyopia), that I realized why.

Thus, in order to cope with presbyopia, I had to have my eyes examined for a lens prescription. This revealed that I also had astigmatism. I must have had it all my life, but when I was young my brain adapted to it so I could see without problems. It was only when I was given spectacles for presbyopia that I became unable to see clearly unless the lenses were also corrected for the astigmatism. I suspect that when I was a medical student, looking through a microscope lens may also have revealed that astigmatism, and as a result the brain was not able to handle the microscope images. This may have been why I was more interested in other ways of investigating anatomies.

When I was much older, I had my astigmatic correction added to the eye-pieces of my binoculars. This meant that, for the first time, I could read the numbers on race horses!

So, in the beginning, I always looked to numbers rather than pictures for investigating anatomies. But even here there were limitations. The old ways of finding numbers were tedious in the extreme, and also limiting. Instruments included rulers, callipers, osteometric boards, scales, and many other *ad hoc* pieces of equipment (such as goniometers for measuring angles), which had already been standard for anatomists and anthropologists for centuries. Measurements were also standard, like length, breadth and thickness, taken from standardized anatomical points. The old studies used numbers in their raw form (size) or modified them as combinations of two measurements (ratios or angles, proportions).

But by my time, such instruments and measurements did not seem to give much new information! They could be bettered. I was lucky enough to come into research quite close to the start of new ways of measuring and new ways of analyzing. These involved borrowing (stealing!) from other disciplines, other colleagues, and other technologies.

Doing Better With Numbers

It was obvious that measurements in one dimension could be improved by making them in two or even three dimensions.

There had been early attempts to do this, as in stereometrics. In particular, in his sadly shortened life, Norman Creel (a colleague, then at Stony Brook) obtained such data by adapting (borrowing, stealing) from geography, the technology for map-making from aerial photography. His equipment was very large, complex and expensive, but it worked!

I myself thought I had a good solution when I came across a piece of equipment called the 'Graf pen'. It was a great idea. The tip of a sound-emitting 'pointer' could project sound to three linear microphones arranged at right angles. These recorded the three-dimensional coordinates of the tip. The sonic data were then converted digitally and displayed in a 'window'. The numbers then had to be copied and punched onto IBM cards for computer analysis (much scope for error!). It worked well for big bones, but was not accurate enough for small bones.

Since then, however, technologies have moved on, through online digital callipers that can put data directly into computers to handling computational measurements from optical and x-ray imaging, to CAT scans and MRIs, and allowing for the ability to rotate bones showing all sides, and even insides. Three-dimensional printing has been invented and this can cope with many problems (e.g., defining the complexity of the spongy network in a bone). These methods came too late for me, but not for my younger colleagues and today's students.

New ways of examining numbers were also needed: statistical analysis and hypothesis testing. Again, these new ways were not, at first, mine. I first learnt simple statistics: means, variances, standard errors, fiducial limits, and significances, with Eric Ashton in Birmingham.

My schoolboy slide rule was not much good for this. So, I first used a Facit, a calculating machine where the motive power for turning the numbered dials was my hand turning a handle. I then graduated to the Monroe and Friden calculators. These were also mechanical calculators, but the motive power for turning the dials was electrical.

I have never forgotten my first 'argument' with a Monroe. I attempted a calculation and the machine started off alright, clicking away. But it went on, and on, and on; it didn't stop! I hit what I thought was the stop key, but it continued on. I looked around surreptitiously to make sure no one had seen what had happened.

In somewhat of a panic, I hit various keys, more or less at random. The machine continued to click! I looked around again to see if anyone had noticed. Then I turned it off at the wall, and the clicking stopped.

I turned it on again, and the clicking again started! I did this twice more: same result. I turned it off and went for a long coffee. When I came back and turned it on, it started clicking again! I turned it off and went home.

It was OK the next day! Of course, I had accidentally divided by zero.

Helped by New Colleagues: Statisticians

When Zuckerman saw that I was really interested in numbers rather than images, he insisted that I meet with real statisticians.

He had, himself, been criticized in public by R. A. Fisher in the 1930s for presenting a paper with means but without any assessment of variation. That kind of public criticism can result in lifelong enmities. This might have been so here because, on the basis of Fisher's comments at the presentation, the abstract of the presentation was rejected for publication! The Physiological Society did that in those days.

However, instead of annoyance, anger, or lifelong enmity, Zuckerman's reaction was to go to Fisher the very next day to find out what he should have done. As a result, Zuckerman was *gung ho* on measurement, analysis and hypothesis testing. (And he used them with great success later during World War II, see another chapter.)

He sent me to see that same Fisher at Rothamstead Experimental Station. Fisher was very nice to me, but he quickly sent me to his 'young man' Yates (who wasn't really young, even then). Frank Yates, just as quickly, sent me to his 'young man' Michael Healey (who really was almost as young as me). Thus, was I introduced to the computer at Rothamstead (was it called the Elliot 409?) and to computer programming in binary code (one makes enormous numbers of errors, and debugging is a PAIN).

Later I graduated to Mercury Autocode (half way between binary code and later computer languages) on the English Electric KDF9 computer in Birmingham.

Later still, as the computers evolved, so did my anatomical studies. Thus, using yet other computers, I started to 'speak' FORTRAN, then COBOL, PASCAL, and so on. I was even interviewed by a reporter who wrote an article on the evolution of the computer for studying the evolution of life.

I was present on one occasion with Yates in Rothamstead when Michael Healy came in and showed him a very large matrix (41×41!) that he had calculated using hand machines. It had taken him several weeks. Yates looked at it and circled three entries.

"Go back and check these."
Healy checked them and they were wrong!
He spent another few weeks redoing the whole matrix. He was furious. Those three were the only ones that were wrong!

Of course, I now know how Yates did it; he squinted at the matrix through half shut eyes. If you look at any large pattern like this, elements that are out of place sometimes stand out. I have done this myself in assessing student results. The students are mystified.

I have (I am half-ashamed to say) often played games like this on students. I have never forgotten when I first obtained a Wang desk computer. It had an additional large box that could perform 8×8 matrix operations. Each cell of the matrix was represented by a light on the side of the box. When matrix operations were in process, the various lights would flicker on and off as numbers went from one cell to another. I was the very picture of the mad scientist. The students were entranced.

However, the Wang was linked to a typewriter through a solenoid so that one could print results. It also had two small punched card readers. A program could start on one card, go through loops on the second card, return to the first, and back to the second, and so on, until the task was complete, allowing the repetitive calculations of statistics.

This was how I first drew sine-cosine waves from minus π to plus π. The program took about two minutes to do the calculation for the first point at minus π. The typewriter would then clunk into life and print an X for the first point on the sine-cosine curve. This was then repeated, taking another two minutes for the second point, and so on until about two hours later the typewriter had printed out the entire wave of Xs from $-\pi$ to $+\pi$.

What a way to do it compared with the present day! The students were entranced again.

They were even more entranced when, as they came to use the Wang themselves, they found that whenever they made certain mistakes, the typewriter would spring into life and type out 'damn, damn, damn'. They never did find out how it happened.

They never noticed the little wire that went from the Wang to an almost-closed drawer in my bench. Hidden in there was a third card reader plus the card that, when activated by the mistake, made the typewriter print out 'damn, damn, damn'!

This statistical collaboration and consultation with Fisher's group in the UK was later continued with Paul Meier, David Wallace and Bill Kruskal when I arrived at the University of Chicago.

Many others, however, also helped the more generally mathematical sides of my work. In Birmingham, Roger Flynn rescued me from more than one statistical error.

Later at Chicago, Joel Cohen (who almost immediately left for Harvard) helped me with multivariate statistics. Peter Neeley, also in Chicago (who almost as quickly left for Kansas), introduced me to his neighborhood limited classification. D. F. Andrews (though I never met him personally) of Bell Telephone Labs (as it was in those days) provided me with his minimum spanning tree program (which he had developed to find the minimum amount of telephone cables to connect cities). In developing this, he used some of our measurements on ape teeth. L. A. Zadeh provided early thoughts about the use of fuzzy sets in understanding biological relationships. Rebecca German, then an undergraduate student at Chicago (but a mathematics major doing undergraduate research with me), and graduate student Gene Albrecht helped me with multivariate statistics.

I, in my turn, was 'used' by others. Business Professor Daryl Bock had me talk to his graduate classes because my data, being 'hard' (i.e., in millimetres), were so much clearer than the 'soft' data from the questionnaires used in his students' business studies. It was easier for his graduate students to differentiate between artefacts due to problems with data as compared with those due to problems with statistics.

Dentist and Professor Tom Graber, whose graduate students were in the Zoller Dental Clinic, was likewise happy to have me talk to his research students about my use of multivariate statistics (in my studies of the shoulder and hip).

I imagine these may be the only times that graduate students in business and dentistry, respectively, have ever heard about the anatomy of shoulders and hips!

Since then, statistical influences from others have continued to be important. In Los Angeles, Gene Albrecht, Bruce Gelvin and Susan Sima Lieberman carried out multivariate analyses on my primate data. In Western Australia, Norm Campbell (CSIRO) helped me through his extension of the original Blackith and Reyment text *Multivariate Morphometrics*, and Adrian Baddeley (Applied Mathematics, University of Western Australia) contributed to Willem de Winter's and my studies of brain data.

Even more recently during retirement, I have been helped by colleagues at the University of York, UK (especially Paul O'Higgins, but also some of his colleagues, e.g., Andrea Cardini, now in Italy, Michael Fagan, University of Hull, UK, and others).

Paul O'Higgins and I wrote a paper only recently on possible additions to his geometric morphometric tool-kit. This raised such violent discussion between the two of us (I thought we were going to have a 'domestic') that we turned to another mathematical colleague, Fred Bookstein, for resolution. I had known Fred for years, as long ago as his PhD studies in the 1970s and the Chicago connection, and through him I came to know the whole group of workers associated with the University of Vienna.

I have, thus, always been blessed by having colleagues gifted in various areas of mathematics, physics and engineering, who were able to help with my biological problems.

Helped With New Data: Gifted, Not Stolen!

In addition to analytical help, I have always been blessed by colleagues were willing to gift me their raw data. This is unusual.

Academics often hide data!

Such colleagues included: Francoise Jouffroy of Paris, who gave me her data on prosimians (as they were called in those days); Brian Johnson of Leeds, UK, who provided radiographs of human vertebrae; Adolf Schultz of Zurich, who gave me his raw data on primate body dimensions; Heinz Stephan of the Max Plank Institute, who gave his unpublished data (individual specimen measures) of brain-part sizes in more than a thousand mammals; Wu Ru Kang of the Academia Sinica, Beijing, who gave his dimensions of literally thousands of fossil teeth; and Pan Ruliang of China and Australia, who shared with me measures of many primate skulls.

Design of Observations: 'Borrowed' From Fisher!

Most important of all to me was Sir Ronald Aylmer Fisher and especially his 1935 book, *The Design of Experiments*. In his introduction, Fisher points out that, for example, the authoritative assertion:

"their controls are totally inadequate"

had been used by many reviewers to discredit many a promising line of work.

Fisher showed that far more information can be obtained by comparing among and between many different experimentals and controls, rather than by single control/experimental pairs. His work was in agriculture where experimentals and controls could be arranged along a *row* of plants in a field. He called these 'Latin squares' (because he used the Latin a, b, c … to designate the various agricultural treatments).

He immediately elaborated this into experimental designs that he called Graeco-Latin Squares (because a second layer of plots at right angles to the first were designated by the terms, α, β, γ …). One can readily see these as *rows of rows* of plants in a field.

The Graeco-Latin squares could be further followed by what Fisher called 'higher squares' where the plots might be in three dimensions (as it were). Thus, a third set of squares might be designated as 1, 2, 3, … and so on, giving a design as of a *cube of rows, of rows, of rows*. I visualized these as stacked cages in an animal house. There could be even more dimensions in the computer. Of course, in real life it may be difficult to actually arrange studies precisely like this.

But Fisher's key point was that enormously more information can be obtained from such combined designs than can possibly be obtained from the very commonly used (in biology and especially medicine) simple experimental/control pairs. The 'squares' clarify complex combinatorial situations, and biology and medicine are complex.

I totally accepted Fisher's exposition. I had not realized that the control/experimental pair (that I learnt in medical school) could be bettered.

But of course, I, and many other workers, did not use experiments. We used observations. I wondered: was a set of observations like a set of experiments?

It was, thus, that I started to think of the comparisons of biological structures in the light of a *design of observations*. Could this, in a parallel way to the *design of experiments*, elucidate observations (especially observations described by numbers)?

Many observational studies in my area of primatology examined structural differences in a pair of species that differed in a specific functional way (e.g., the differences in anatomies of two species showing lesser and greater degrees of arboreality, or lesser and greater degrees of leaping, etc). Of course, though the difference between the members of such a pair might well relate to the functional difference, it might well also relate to something completely different. Thus, this is a weak comparison (even if it appears strong when of high statistical significance).

But, like Fisher's design of experiments, how much more powerful is a design of observations contrasting several species that differ in a linear sequence? Such a study might examine linear sequences of several species of, say, cercopithecine monkeys that inhabit, serially:

(a) terrestrial niches,
(b) semi-terrestrial niches,
(c) the arboreal main branch, and
(d) arboreal fine branch niches.

Another example might be the comparison of several species of, say, bush babies involved serially in:

(a) less leaping,
(b) more leaping,
(c) highly leaping, and
(d) extreme leaping.

Any relationships consistent within such **one-dimensional linear designs** [(a) through (d) in both examples] are much more likely to give functional results implied in the functional descriptions than single simple pair-wise comparisons.

A second level of observational design, perhaps rather more difficult to obtain, but with even further power, involves the use of **two-dimensional parallel (as it were) designs**.

Thus, studies of differences in climbing in Old World monkeys might include serial comparison of several pairs of linear designs:

more terrestrial (a'), less terrestrial (a") and least terrestrial (a''') cercopitheque monkeys;
more terrestrial (b'), less (b') and least (b''') mangabeys;
more terrestrial (c'), less (c") and least (c''') macaques; and
more terrestrial (d'), less (d") and least (d''') langurs.

Such parallel (two-dimensional) designs give even more power in detecting differences among the species related to the functional differences posited.

A third level of observations could combine these in **three-dimensional comparisons** within the same group of animals:

more (a'), less (a"), less still (a''') and least (a'''') leaping **colobines**, more (b'), less (b"), less still (b''') and least (b'''') arboreal **colobines** and,
more (c'), less (c"), less still (c''') and least (c'''') high altitude **colobines**, with

the same series of

(a'...'s)
(b'...'s) and
(c'...'s) **macaques**

and the same series of

(a'...'s)
(b'...'s) and
(c'...'s) **cercopitheques**.

Of course, it might well be difficult to obtain the full suite of possibilities. Some 'cells' might have to be empty.

In these examples, my *design of observations* of monkeys mimics Fisher's *design of experiments* of plants, even resembling his Latin, Graeco-Latin and higher squares.

They helped me disentangle effects truly due to functional, behavioral and environmental parallels from effects due to hereditary, phylogenetic or even just random baggage. This does not mean it is wrong to compare only pairs of species. But these multiple combinations are much more powerful and make much more use of data than pairs. In addition, merely thinking about such design possibilities sharpened the mind about the real questions being examined. In this way 'Fisher' became my 'God'.

Of course, Gods sometimes have feet of clay!

Further Design of Observations: 'Stolen' From McCloskey!

In the 1970s, I met Donald McCloskey when he was being interviewed for a college appointment in Chicago. In retrospect, I am so pleased that I supported his appointment. But the real significance of this was not clear to me until 50 years later when we met at a symposium in the Konrad Lorenz Institute, Altenburg, Austria.

That meeting first produced the usual exchange: What university were you at? For both of us it was the University of Chicago. During what years? For both of us it was in the 1970s. Did we know each other? It turned out that I, as Dean, had interviewed him for an appointment.

But of course, in 2011, I was talking to Deidre McCloskey. Donald had undergone gender reassignment, and Deidre was happy in her new role. Eleanor and I were delighted for her!

More important to this story is the fact that Deidre had published, in 2008, a book with Stephen T. Ziliak titled *The Cult of Statistical Significance*. It is a marvelous book pointing out that, however important many of the earlier statistics were in the social and life sciences, they were also capable of being mishandled in ways that 'Student' (William Sealy Gosset), the inventor of the 't' test, always warned that they would be.

"Fit,"
Gosset said,
"is not the same thing as importance. Statistical significance is not the same thing as scientific finding."

Though the importance of Fisher's design of experiments can scarcely be overestimated, it must be used with a sense of how 'real significance' can transform many problems.

The mainstream in science, as any scientist should tell you, is sometimes wrong. Otherwise, come to think of it, science would be almost complete. Few scientists would make that claim, or would want to. Yet the conventional wisdom, especially strong the further we are from animals and the closer we are to humans, can be extremely difficult to change.

In many fields (social and biological sciences, human sciences and medicine), the idol — *the gold standard* — is the test of significance (whether through a simple univariate 't' test calculated almost on the fingers, or a complex multivariate statistic derived by machine computations not always understood by the worker). I, myself, value statistics as crucial.

But one part of statistics has gone wrong. Reducing the scientific problem of measurement, testing and interpretation to one of 'statistical significance', as many of us have done for almost one hundred years, has sometimes been a bad idea. Significance, reduced to its narrow meaning only, may have little to do with rational decision making.

One problem here is that the qualitative answer, *yes or no*, may hide the quantitative answer, such as how much is the effect or how many different effects are there.

In other words, we do not want a simple answer (in black or white). We want a complex answer that encompasses many (but hopefully not 50) shades of grey.

We do not want an answer that says: this **is** the diagnosis; for example, this **is** a new species — **or not** — full stop. We want an answer that recognizes that there is a spectrum of possible answers; some we may expect, some may be unexpected, and some may be totally in left field! Vital answers may be dismissed or overlooked because they were hidden in the blind spot of the preconceived idea, in the tyranny of the false dichotomy.

Should we be distinguishing technical significance testing from real hypothesis testing?

Trespassing: From Description to Interpretation

My initial uses of statistics were aimed at trying to compare forms. Quickly, however, they came to suggest possibilities for the interpretation of forms.

This started with my dissatisfaction with the method of anatomical inference, the main way in which function was inferred (or better: 'guessed') from form. Not that functional inference is inherently bad; it's just that there are better ways of understanding the function/structure duality, particularly in the muscle/bone/joint mechanism.

So, I took a practical course on experimental stress and strain analysis at the Royal College of Advanced Technology at Salford (now the University of Salford).

The lecturers on that course were partly amused and partly horrified by having one student who turned up with wet and bloody (but not warm) bones, instead of oily crankshafts. I wanted to apply strength of materials to bone and bones.

One technique involved comparing (through a microscope) a grid inscribed upon an object with the same grid after straining the object. It worked with metals; not well with bones.

Another technique was to compare grids shadowed on objects of different shape through the moiré fringes that appear when the grids are superimposed. Again, this is not a matter of actual mechanical strains. It gives geometric 'strains' involved in 'pretending' that one bone shape has become changed ('strained') into the other.

Yet a third direction involved examining the cracks produced in a lacquer coating on the surface of an object when loaded. Real mechanical strains cause these cracks. I never actually did this on bones, though others did. It involved cyanide for annealing the lacquers and seemed just too dangerous in my unsophisticated hands.

And a fourth used the property of photoelasticity. Certain transparent materials, especially many plastics, rotate the plane of polarized light when they are strained. The beginnings of this technique were in the 1820s (by Brewster, the father; a famous name in 19th century science). No plastics then; Brewster used glass! Of course, glass is so insensitive that it only shows perhaps one-third of a fringe before breaking under load. How many models did Brewster break? Even the broken models led to advances because, as a result, he invented techniques for multiplying the number of fringes before breaking. By my time plastics had been invented, and some were exceedingly sensitive.

Accordingly, a plastic model of a bone can, when strained, give some information about strain. Of course, only the model is strained, not the bone, and it was only two-dimensional. One reviewer denigrated this as my playing with *"little plastic cut-outs!"*

I then met Ken Sharples of Sharples PhotoLasticity Inc., bought his polariscope (Figure 7.1) and applied it to the mechanics of scapular form.

The method was applied to the femoral head with a prosthesis in place (Figure 7.2). Even though simplistic, this showed that the prosthesis was badly designed because it markedly increased strain at a certain point in the model. Of course, the surgeons already knew that, because patients had been coming back with a small fracture at exactly that point.

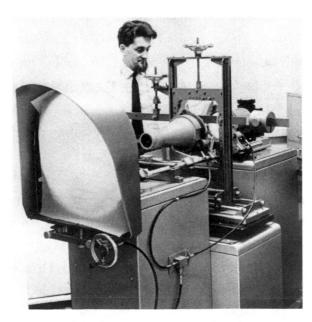

Figure 7.1:   The Sharples polariscope.

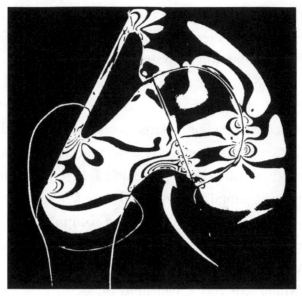

Figure 7.2: Two-dimensional photoelastic model of the femoral head and neck with a piece shaped like a prosthesis. The white arrow shows the many lines where stresses are large!

The photoelastic idea was further extended when, on a day when I was bored, I was casually turning over the pages of a number of the *Journal of the Aeronautical Society* in the academic staff common room in Birmingham. My eyes lit upon an article:

"An Experimental Stress Analysis of Aircraft Landing Gear".

My immediate and almost irreverent reaction was:

"If aircraft landing gear, why not monkey landing gear?"

This led me to Westland's Aircraft Ltd. It was in the Isle of Wight, close to Southampton where my father had worked on the Spitfire at Supermarine Works before the war.

I bought their reflection polariscope, which allowed me to visualize strains in bones through strains in a thin photoelastic coating applied to the surface of the bone. Loading the bone then not only strained the bone but also strained the coating which, because of its photoelastic properties, became birefringent.

Whereas the simpler Sharples polariscope described above examined two-dimensional models of the shape of a bone, the Westlands Aircraft reflection polariscope showed the real strains in the photoelastic coating produced by the real surface strains on the three-dimensional bone (Figures 7.3 and 7.4). This still meant that loadings were very simplistic compared to what must happen in life.

Stress and strain analyses today use computational finite elements. They model objects by representing them as many small elements, each one of which gives strains at its locus. Summing them over whole structures gives field views.

At first, in the 1970s with a graduate student (Artyan Hsu) in physical therapy at the University of Southern California, we did this two-dimensionally on radiographs of the human heel bone. It was at 'toe off' in walking that the largest strains are encountered, and that it is to these strains that the internal structure is most closely related (Figure 7.5).

Commercial Reflection Polariscope

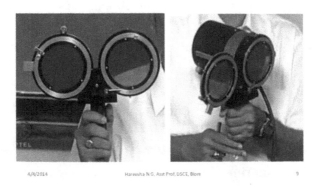

Figure 7.3:   The reflection polariscope.

P. S. Testing under progress on a main landing gear of Airbus A 330/A340 passenger air craft

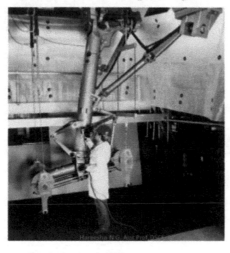

Figure 7.4: The reflection polariscope's use for looking at aircraft landing gear, but not, of course, from the original paper that I saw — this one was much later — but the method is still in use.

Previously, it had been thought that 'heel strike' provided the highest strains. The very words 'heel strike' seem to say that. Today, the importance of toe-off is well accepted. It has led to better ways of running and better architectures for running shoes.

More finite element studies followed after my move to the University of Western Australia. The work with the UK group continued, but I also met with new colleagues in geomechanics (Chris Windsor and Wayne Robertson from the geomechanics unit of the CSIRO), who introduced me to more modern elements of finite element analysis performed with fast lagrangian analysis of continua (FLAC). Research assistant Christine Runnion (previously from Liverpool University where she had worked with Bernard Wood) and I used FLAC to study patterns in human vertebral bodies.

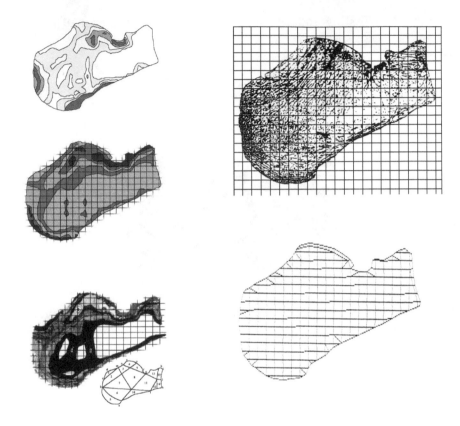

Figure 7.5:   Left three frames: strains at heel strike (upper), mid-stance (middle) and toe off (lower). Right two frames: the close association between stress pattern and bone pattern is at toe off.

This collaboration led to the smallest research grant I have ever had (a one-year pilot grant of $17,000), which allowed me to pay Christine Runnion. I am proud of it as it was awarded by a 'modern engineering funding agency' to an 'old fashioned medical anatomist'!

Further collaborations followed with Paul O'Higgins (then with us at UWA) before he moved to a professorship at University College London, and later as the Founding Professor of anatomy at the Universities of York and Hull, UK.

Now such studies are carried out in York and in Hull, mostly by Professors Paul O'Higgins, Michael Fagan, Catherine Dobson, Kornelius Kupczik, and many other colleagues, and especially using three-dimensional developments (Figure 7.6).

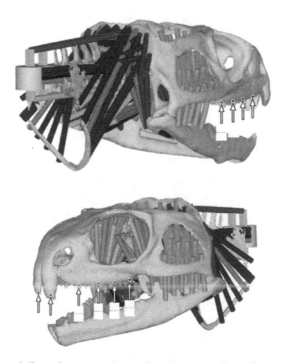

Figure 7.6: Modelling chewing and muscle actions on a three-dimensional rendering of the muscles and bones in a skull (courtesy of Prof. Michael Fagan).

More Borrowing: From Patterns to Textures

My initial 1950s interests in the external form of bones led to almost equally early (1960s) interests in the internal textures of bones. In biology, they were firstly introduced as 'morphometrics' for studying the patterns revealed by the microscope.

But these were not satisfactory to me; the methods were called morphometrics, but with a meaning completely different from the morphometrics in *multivariate morphometrics*. They required expensive instruments that, in those days, were financially impossible for a single investigator. Much cheaper and much better ways of understanding complex textures were already being used outside anatomy.

Some came from psychologists interested in problems of vision (Harold Blum), from geologists interested in rock patterns (John Davis), from astronauts and astronomers at NASA interested in pictures taken in space, from the defence industry examining aerial photographs, and today from many, many others.

And some were, of course, classified.

I have never forgotten being asked by Solly Zuckerman (at the time that he was Chief Adviser on Science and Defence to the UK Government) to describe the work I was then doing. His response:

> *"That's all very interesting, but the people working in*
> *defence are way ahead.*
> *I cannot tell you about it, the work is classified!"*

I started to 'borrow' a variety of these techniques. I borrowed 'medial axis transforms' from Harold Blum, who invented them for looking at visual fields. Of course, he was looking at the retina, which was not flat but curved. I used it to look at the curved surface of the pelvis (Figure 7.7).

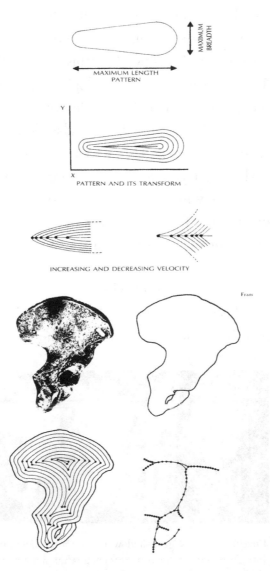

Figure 7.7:   Upper frames: Blum's methods of characterizing a shape through the medial axis transform. Lower frames: applying Blum's method to the three-dimensional hip bone.

In turn, Waddington borrowed from me in 1977, picking up my usage in his fascinating book, *Tools for Thought*.

I then borrowed another method employing moiré fringes. This involved shadowing a grid upon a plane, and then superimposing that grid upon the grid distorted by being shadowed on an object. This produced moiré fringes reflecting the true three-dimensionality of the object. Figure 7.8 shows how this works with a pelvis.

Next, I became involved in geological pattern recognition. This occurred because Dr. Peter Neeley (who, in Chicago, had introduced me to neighborhood limited classification) had moved to the University of Kansas. He introduced me to the geologist John Davis, who was trying to understand patterns in oil-bearing rock sections. I knew instantly that this would be good for sections and radiographs of bones. The method used an optical bench and a laser to produce optical Fourier transforms (this was before computational fast Fourier transforms). John printed for me the first color transforms of a vertebral section.

Later I took a course given by Harry Pincus of the University of Wisconsin at Milwaukee. He had taken the idea of John Davis'

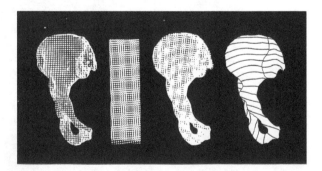

Figure 7.8:   First frame: a flat grid shadowed upon a hip bone; next frame: two flat grids differing by a few degrees shadowed on each other showing moiré fringes; third frame: a flat grid laid across the grid in the first frame showing the moiré fringes due to the three-dimensional shape of the hip bone; fourth frame: lines describing the three-dimensionality of the hip bone.

optical bench (22 feet long) and folded it with mirrors into a small box ($2 \times 2 \times 2$ feet).

The power of this technology is shown by examining the lateral radiographs of vertebral bodies. The overwhelming visual impression in the radiograph is a right-angled network. But the transform shows that, in addition, there are many bony spicules at other angles that are important in helping us understand how cancellous bones bear loads (Figure 7.9).

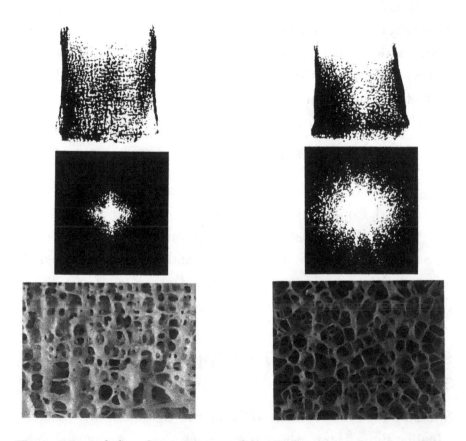

Figure 7.9: Left three frames: First, a radiograph of a vertebra showing, visually, a right-angled pattern of bony spicules. Second, the optical Fourier transform, cruciate in form, confirms the visual impression. Third, confirmed by the pattern in an actual section. Right three frames: First, a radiograph of another vertebra seemingly also showing a general right-angled pattern. Second, its star-like Fourier transform, implying material lying in many different directions. Third, the Fourier transform is correct.

In my readings about Fourier transforms, I also came across other transforms such as the Haar, Hadamard, Walsh and Hadamard-Walsh transforms. They were all being used to examine textures in pictures: the form of leaves in botany, earliest moon shots from the surveyor space craft, and classified data from military aerial photographs.

I was reading about these transforms and becoming more and more puzzled. This was because I am mathematically illiterate.

It took me a year to realize their mathematical relationships. They are all part of a single overarching series called the Karhunen-Loeve series (named after Kari Karhunen and Michel Loeve). Moreover, I gradually learnt that they are related to principal components, canonical variates and Hotelling (multivariate) analyses, already all known to me as elements of multivariate statistics.

A real mathematician knows these things almost instinctively.

Eventually however, even optical Fourier transforms were superceded. Computational Fourier transforms came along.

For me this was set up by a programmer, Roger Sweetman, who wrote the software 'fluffy puppy', and my graduate research assistant, later my doctoral student and now Dr. Alanah Buck, forensic anthropologist, who carried out the analyses (Figure 7.10).

Serendipity (A Word That Appears Many Times in This book)

Serendipity of this kind has so frequently figured in my research. Meeting René Thom, who was giving a series of seminars (1960s) at the University of Chicago, introduced me to catastrophe theory. His ideas stayed with me but only came to fruition some

Females   Males

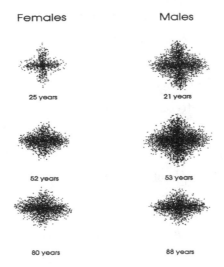

Figure 7.10: Computational Fourier transforms of vertebral sections of six exemplar individuals, three males and three females. The cruciate forms of the transform indicate primarily right-angled textures in young females and young males: no osteoporosis. The rugby football shapes of the transforms in the oldest males and females show a loss of that right-angled texture as in osteoporosis in both sexes. However, the middle-aged males still show the right-angled texture but the middle-aged females the rugby football texture. Hence osteoporosis is present in the middle-aged females but not the middle-aged males!

50 years later. Like the artistic beginnings of D'Arcy Thompson's coordinate transformations (from Albert Durer's transformations of faces in the 17th century), it had, for me, an artistic conclusion in Salvatore Dalī's work at the end of the 20th century (see earlier figures).

I don't know where I got the idea of borrowing (hopefully not stealing) from workers and disciplines. Nevertheless, I could enthusiastically share methodological toolkits with those from many other branches of knowledge, especially the mathematical, physical and engineering sciences, disciplines in which I have almost no grounding at all. It was fascinating to find commonalities.

These commonalities led, in combination, to new themes. Thus, from the 'mathematical arrangements of monkeys by anatomies', I was able to fashion another seemingly opposite theme, 'the mathematical arrangement of anatomies by monkeys'! The first of these seemed to be an expression of function, the second an expression of development. These ideas have led on to combined studies that seem to provide an interplay between function and development with implications for evolution.

It sometimes frightens me to realize how many of these new technologies, new collaborations, and new colleagues seem to have been totally serendipitous.

Further, I especially worry about how many even better techniques I, myself, have missed because of the individuals, the places, and the ideas that I did NOT encounter.

Further again, I have used these new technologies to take delight in pointing out both the complexity of what has generally been rejected as simple, and the simplicity of what is sometimes viewed as hopelessly complex.

Serendipity can, in fact, be generated: by reading in others' disciplines, attending others' seminars, discussing science at coffee time, taking seminars and courses in other institutions, attending to scientific papers outside one's own area, and so on. Yet it is so hard to get graduate students to go to seminars apparently outside their own problems.

Nevertheless, the people who have contributed most to my research over the years, indeed, the people who keep me mentally alive even now, are my own graduate students. Many of them, now professors in their turn, in all parts of the world, and, in turn, their students, and not a few of their students' students, are 'still mine'!

Some are now 'retired'. How frightening still that even one of my student's students is retired!

It is through all these individuals that I am still able to be involved in new developments. They keep me alive. They are the ones I honor. They are present in spirit as I look at my seventy years in science and medicine, and as I contemplate the further years (I hope) in which I will continue to be involved as an honorary investigator, during which my ideas may help yet further generations of science and medical students.

8 Three Heresies and Thrice a Heretic!

Though in other chapters I have emphasized the importance of loyalty to people, disciplines and institutions, in research there can be misplaced loyalty to ideas.

We Are Not Always Right!

We need to check our ideas and root out our mistakes (quite difficult). We must do this even if the ideas seem inimical to the conventional wisdom (this is more difficult). And we must especially do this even if the ideas destroy our own most ardently held notions (this is most difficult of all). Research is neither a matter of counting votes, nor a matter of the will of the majority. One fact that destroys a hypothesis is stronger than a hundred that support it.

Research is not a list of successes; we make mistakes all the time. As Mario Livio wrote:

"The road to triumph is paved with blunders."

In contrast, Linus Pauling said:

"Mistakes do no harm in science because there are lots of smart people out there who will immediately spot a mistake and correct it."

Unfortunately, Pauling was not right. Some scientists, sometimes many scientists, support ideas because of prior views. The power of prior views, and of the scientists who own them, to prevent advance is great!

Thus:
How do we decide when to give up an idea which many aver is a dead end?
How do we persevere with a 'dead' idea, to discover it was not dead after all?
How do we discard a conventional idea, to be able to propose a new?
In trying to work out such matters, I have been an academic heretic many times.

Though I first studied the bones of today's monkeys, apes and humans, it was always with fossils in mind. Yet I was well aware of the 'FFF', or fossil finders' fights.

I was afraid of FFF! This was why I worked first on the shoulder blade, a bone so fragile and so easily damaged that it is almost never found as a fossil. This meant I would not be disputing someone else's fossil.

This policy worked.

Thus, I found that the form of the human shoulder, even among the wide array of shoulders of many other living mammals, was unique. This can be seen from the position for the human shoulder amongst the large cloud of points representing the shoulders of other mammals (Figure 8.1).

Because a fossil was not involved, the work was well accepted.

In contrast, the next bone I worked on was the hip. This bone is bigger and stronger than the shoulder blade and, as a result,

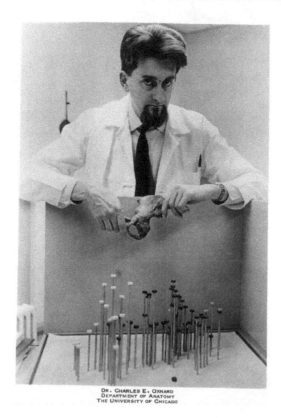

Figure 8.1: The old way (see a young Oxnard above) of demonstrating three-dimensional results: not a computer-drawn plot, but a physical model. The small separate dot below is the human shoulder. (The photographer made me hold a pelvis — it was bigger!)

more frequently found as a reasonably complete fossil. It was almost inevitable that I would run into trouble.

Therefore, A First Heresy: Walking on Two Legs

The trouble came because a fairly complete fossil hip bone was already known. Though australopithecine skulls were largely ape-like, the australopithecine pelvis was alleged to be part-way to human and therefore indicated human bipedalism and, hence, a human ancestor!

This was the conventional wisdom.

Our work challenged this.

We found that this pelvis was not part-way between four-limbed climbing apes and two-legged bipedal humans. Rather, it differed from both in a triangular relationship. It certainly was not a simple intermediate (Figure 8.2).

This figure shows that the fossil has a triangular relationship to humans and apes, and is not intermediate! That idea was anathema in those days. And indeed, even today, there are still many who hold to the idea that these fossils were bipedal, even fully bipedal, and therefore direct intermediaries to humans.

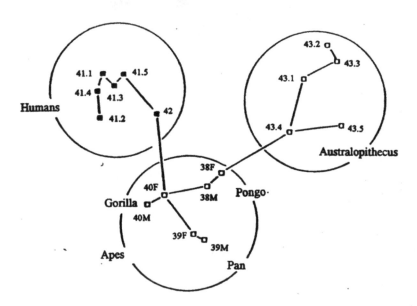

Figure 8.2:   Hip bones in modern apes, modern humans and *Australopithecus* as seen in a similar analysis as used in Figure 8.1. The positions of five different attempts at reconstructing the australopithecine hip are shown.

This Heresy Has Long Roots

This heresy (for heresy it was) started with Solly Zuckerman more than a hundred years ago, before he had left South Africa.

Sitting at a bench doing research (though just a medical student!), he overheard a discussion between his head of department in Cape Town University, Professor M. R. Drennan, and a visiting colleague, Raymond Dart, newly appointed Professor in the University of Witwatersrand. They were trying to decide if a skull they were examining was a baby gorilla or a baby chimpanzee. Zuckerman realized they could not tell which was which!

Yet in spite of this indecision over these two complete identified living specimens, Dart had no hesitation in asserting, and Drennan in accepting, that the partial and somewhat distorted newly found fossil baby skull (the 'Taung Baby') was pre-human!

Many years later, Zuckerman returned to the question of human evolutionary origins. By then more fossils had been unearthed in South Africa, and later East Africa. All were similarly hailed as 'missing links' in human ancestry, intermediates on an evolutionary pathway from earlier ape-like species to later human-like forms. These conclusions reminded Zuckerman of his experience of Dart's and Drennan's certainty about the humanness of the incomplete Taung baby in the light of their uncertainty about complete ape babies.

At this later stage, whenever Zuckerman checked information about skull form, he found two things. First, some features of australopithecines really were more like living humans; these were features that were always emphasized in the conventional certainty about their pre-humanness. Second, other features of australopithecines more resembled living apes, and these were features that were de-emphasized in their assessment as pre-human.

Of course, even though various humans and apes differ among themselves, all have many features in which they are similar. After all, all humans and all apes are in the same overarching group.

Therefore, Zuckerman was cautious about accepting these 'ex cathedra' pronouncements. Many people misinterpreted this caution as the heresy of him saying that the fossils were just some ape. That was not so; his caution was because of his perception that the fossils were uncritically accepted as pre-human; this was his real initial heresy.

But his much greater heresy was to doubt the certainty involved in this and many other such anthropological judgments.

Our raw data on the pelvic bone were not dissimilar to those on skulls. They, too, showed some measures similar to humans, and some similar to apes. But the new statistical methods (taking all measures together) that we used, when applied to the pelvis, showed that the fossil was not intermediate; it was different from both. And this might have different implications for evolution!

Our findings went further, however. They not only seemed to provide evidence about ape-like, human-like, and neither ape-like-nor-human-like elements of hip shape, but they also seemed to provide information about hip function.

Thus, the human-like elements of the fossil were those aspects describing the sacral and hip joints being placed rather close, as in humans. This seemed related to the trunk and lower limbs being used for weight bearing in line on two legs, as in human upright movement.

The ape-like elements of the fossil were those describing the attachments and leverages of muscles being placed like those in modern apes. This seemed related to muscle function in which lower limbs are used at right angles to the trunk, as in modern apes moving on all fours.

The combination of some ape-like and some human-like elements existing together in the fossil implied that it may not have moved like either humans or apes, nor was it intermediate. It may have moved differently from both. Again, this had new implications for the evolutionary relationship!

Our assessment had thus gone from comparing different forms to suggesting different functions. But did it? How could we tell?

Grounds for Doubt

This finding could have meant a combination in the fossil of some of the activities of both humans and apes. But, if so, it would be a combination not found in any one of them and therefore be different from both. For instance, it could be due to the combination in one creature of some kind of bipedal movement somewhat like that of humans, together with quadrupedal and climbing abilities somewhat like those in apes; a first heresy!

But a second possibility could be a set of activities that did not exist in combination in either apes or humans. I asked, tongue in cheek of course, if perhaps these creatures jumped around on their thumbs!

What these results deny, however, is the idea that the fossils were a simple intermediate between apes and humans. *This was the principal heresy!*

> *But the possibility that they may have been doing something different seemed worth chasing.*

Many years later, a student and now colleague, Algis Kuliukas, suggested a uniquely different combination of activities: not a climbing life largely in the trees (like arboreal nonhuman primates), not a quadrupedal life on the ground (like terrestrial nonhuman primates), not bipedal walking and running (like humans), but yet another combination. My original idea had been: perhaps a combination of both ground progression and tree climbing, which I still think is highly likely. Kuliukas' suggestion included something more. Perhaps some combination of ground progression, tree climbing, and *wading at the waterside*. If you've ever heard a heresy, this is it!

It is at certainly true that the fossils were not found in relation to the deep jungle where mainly upper-limb tree-climbing species predominate, nor on wide plains where largely four-limb ground-running species abound. These fossils truly are found in localized regions of bushes and trees in valleys, around rivers and river banks, even alongside lakes and beaches with woodland fringes. Such environments all combine trees, ground and water!

The initial idea arose well before Kuliukas' time. But for many years, it was much denigrated under the earlier title of Elaine Morgan's 'aquatic ape'. Kuliukas has modified it as a 'waterside hypothesis'. Perhaps these creatures were neither solely a forest species nor solely a savannah species, but an isolated, woodland, water-side, species. They lived in all three parts of that environment: able to wade in water, move on the ground, and climb in trees. Deep forest or vast savannah alone, their environment was not! Kuliukas' idea has been recently supported by Sir David Attenborough.

Such a lifestyle combination might render their anatomies different from any ape or any human.

But apart from this special idea, the relationships of these species have another interesting implication: perhaps there had been more than one primate experiment in bipedalism.

Perhaps bipedalism has arisen twice, and if twice, then possibly more. Some would deny this on the basis of Occam's Razor. But in fact, Occam's Razor really says it is the **simplest** idea that is most likely. If something can arise once, it can also arise a number of times, and **this** is the simple idea. It is the **single origination** that is the more complex and therefore more unlikely.

As a result (and with difficulty), I published in *Nature*, with the title 'Australopithecines: Grounds for Doubt'!

The very title was anathema. It was generally assumed that I meant they were just apes.

All of this really implies that the australopithecines were neither: lineal ancestors of modern apes (as some people thought Zuckerman had said), nor
lineal ancestors of modern humans (the conventional story).

They may have lain on their own **separate branch or branches** within a **complex bush** of forms containing apes and pre-apes, humans and pre-humans (and, perhaps, even a number of other species not found as fossils [and therefore with no names] as well). That is, they **may not** be directly related to the apes, but they **may equally not** have given rise to humans. *They may have just become extinct, like most of the species of those days. Further heresy indeed!*

A Different Heresy in This Story!

A final curious element of heresy in this story is how my views about the australopithecines and human evolution have been deliberately misinterpreted as major support for, first, *biblical origins*, then *creation science*, and now *intelligent design!*

And there is no way that I can rid Google or blogs or tweets or Facebook of such rubbish! In truth, in the beginning I didn't even know this rubbish existed because I never found it.

Of course, that was because I always typed in 'Googol', as a good scientist would!

What do colleagues think about this heresy?

Some Collegial Comments

In 2004, Matt Cartmill, then at Duke University, wrote:
"All of these issues are of course still debated. But on every one of these points the current consensus has largely shifted to Oxnard's view of things. Most of the rest of us are just now catching up with the positions that Charles Oxnard took over 25 years ago. That fact has not been sufficiently appreciated."
(Of course, Cartmill was one of my doctoral students in Chicago, so this is not strong support as antagonists would expect that my student would support me!).
But, if you know Matt Cartmill, you would know that he would not have said that just because I was one of his original supervisors!

Twelve years later in 2016, Bernard Wood, in his blog, 'Publications that (should have) made a difference: Thinking out of the box', wrote: "Most of Charles Oxnard's research concerns living primates, but he has made the occasional foray into the analysis of the hominin fossil record and his lengthy review in *Nature* in 1975 (Australopithecines: Grounds for Doubt) deserves more attention than it has received. My prediction is that it will loom much larger in the history of paleoanthropology than its citation history suggests ... it is one of the first papers, if not the first, to say explicitly that 'bipedalism may have arisen more than once' ... [and] ... 'that climbing may have been part of the locomotor repertoire of archaic hominins'."

In this blog, Bernard Wood further recognized that academic antagonisms may get in the way! Thus, Bernard also wrote:
"I was caught between a 'rock' and a 'hard place'. The 'rock' was that I was a graduate student of Michael Day, in the vanguard of advocating that one of the 'australopithecines' (aka *H. habilis*) was a biped practicing a type of bipedalism that could not be distinguished from the bipedalism practiced by modern humans. The 'hard place' consisted of *Oxnard's compelling opposite results* and, later, **the results of my own ... quantitative analyses**.

"But the really radical aspect of Oxnard's review, that does not seem so radical now, but which in 1975 was heretical, was that: the australopithecines must have lain on an evolutionary side branch for a long time.

"A second, even more radical view was that: perhaps as long as five million years ago or even longer ago, there may have been many creatures living that were generally somewhat similar to *Homo erectus* and therefore classifiable as man in a way that we must now deny to *Australopithecus* (whether named "*H. habilis*", "*H. africanus*" or whatever else).

"So, what encouraged Oxnard to adopt these radical ideas?

"Today, there is now compelling evidence that upright bipedalism does have a deep history in the hominin clade. There is also compelling evidence for more than one type of foot and [more than] one type of pelvis, and thus there must be more than one type of bipedalism within the hominin clade. Oxnard's foresight deserves more recognition than it has received."

These thoughts are especially important because, as is evident in his own words, **Wood's academic heritage, in contrast to Cartmill's, means that he 'should have been' on the other side of the fence!**

A Second Heresy: Uniqueness of the Human Brain

From this, my earliest heresy (which may be starting to be accepted), we can move, perhaps, to an intermediate heresy: the uniqueness of the human brain. The overall story is fully documented elsewhere. But the heresy is detailed here.

In the late 1990s, a mature student (Willem de Winter) came to me with a serious problem. His supervisor had, unfortunately, just died. Willem was interested in behavior and the brain, and the work was already started. Would I be willing to help him finish his doctorate on behavioral plasticity? I said I was very interested in his ideas, but that I generally preferred to test ideas with data and analyses.

Willem, in his turn, said he had become very interested in my use of data. He was especially excited when he found that I had not only analyzed anatomical data (morphometrics) but also behavioral data (with two colleagues, Robin Huw Crompton and Susan Sima Lieberman). We had called this study: 'niche-metrics'.

It seemed reasonable to us both that such analyses might be applied to data on brains, with the possibility of revealing something of brain function, behavioral plasticity, and, tongue in cheek as we would call it, 'neurometrics'!

But where would we get data?

In those days, whenever scientists looked at brains, the primary finding was that brain and body size relations differed among several major animal groups (Figure 8.3).

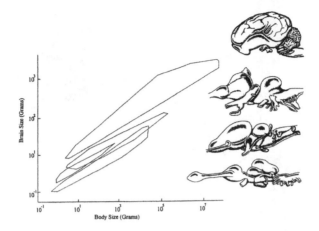

Figure 8.3: Plot of brain size against body size in several different animal groups, from mammals above through birds, reptiles and fishes below, shows different brain/body relationships.

However, for single major groups, there are single straight-line relationships (Figure 8.4).

Surely size could not be all there was in these data?
Could we take this further?

It so happened that Heinz Stephan of the Max Planck Institute had published, over his lifetime, remarkable information about the sizes of eleven brain parts. He had data for more than a thousand specimens representing about 40 species of insectivores, bats and primates (including humans).

Only studies on the 40 species means had ever been published, and it was on these means that most of the literature was based. But with our morphometric techniques, we could include information from all the specimens!

I must here record it as remarkable, even wonderful, that Heinz was willing to give Willem and I these data. Of course, he did not have the techniques that we were proposing. Nevertheless,

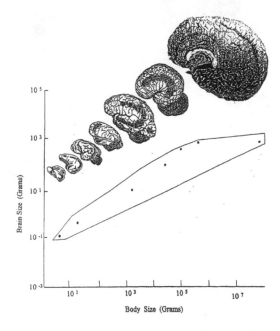

Figure 8.4: Relationship between brain size and body size within primates (but including two very large creatures: the 'honorary primates' of dolphins and whales). Here, there is only one almost straight-line relationship between brain size and body size, and there is nothing special about the place of humans (third brain from the top). It fits completely into the straight line!

it was still a remarkable *gift* (and one of several that I have received during my life, e.g., from Adolph Schultz, Francoise Jouffroy, Wu Ru Kang, Peter Lisowski, Robin Crompton and Pan Ruliang).

We applied our statistics to Stephan's individual brain part sizes. Willem wrote a significant thesis that melded both his original theoretical ideas on brain plasticity and my applied suggestions on brain-part inter-relationships. Ernst Mayr and George Williams were his two distinguished examiners; they rated his work as 'highly commended'. This was even to the point of Mayr accepting Willem's criticisms of some of his (Mayr's) own prior opinions (unusual acceptance indeed, but very welcome).

It was only when we came to publish that we realized we had become heretics.

Surely It Is Not All Just Based on Size?

Of course, many investigators had analyzed Stephan's data on species means using the classical bivariate methods that were pretty much all that were available in earlier times. More recently, however, a few investigators had realized the value of using multivariate statistics. But because the data were only available as 'means of species', the only question they could ask of their multivariate statistics was: *"How are the species means arranged?"*

Principal components analysis, using the 'between the species means' information, could find that answer. The results were always simple. The means were always arranged along a single axis, and were 96% associated with overall body and brain size. The species with the smallest brains lay at one end of the linear array, those with the largest at the other.

Enough said, one would think! Yet our almost irreverent thought was: *"Surely these incredible data (incredibly difficult to obtain) can tell us more than just overall size!"*

Could These Extensive Data Really Tell Us Nothing Else?

Because we had values for every specimen in every species, we could ask a different question:

*"How are the means between the species arranged **when allowance is made for the variations among the specimens within each species?**"*

This question requires a more complex statistical method, so we chose canonical variate analysis which uses both the 'between' and 'within' data matrices.

And we could also ask that question using not only *the simple **raw** sizes of brain parts*, but also *the sizes of brain parts **relative** to one another other*.

That is, while we might expect 'raw brain part sizes' to be mainly about size, we might also expect 'relative brain part sizes' to relate, at least in part, to 'relative functional links' between brain parts.

Of course, we did both. But it was the 'relative' aspect that showed a bold new picture. As a first stab at the 'relative' problem, we looked at the size of each of brain part relative to the size of the main gateway between the body and the brain. We thought this might relate, to some extent at least, to nervous system traffic to and from the body and the brain; *pace* the additional cranial nerve traffic.

But we also thought that perhaps the ratios of the sizes of different individual brain parts to one another might reflect functional cross-talk within the brain. So, we examined, for example, the cerebellum relative to the cerebral cortex, the midbrain relative to the diencephalon, and so on.

In other words, we felt it possible that the *relative sizes* of parts *within the brain* might reflect something of their *functional interactions*.

This is an enormously crude idea compared to what can be done today with CAT scans, PET scans, MRIs, and many even newer techniques that can show function. But these expensive and time-consuming methods are available for humans mostly in medical contexts.

Who in this world could apply them to several tens of nonhuman species and many hundreds of nonhuman specimens: the size of our data set?

And where would they get the specimens and their brains?

And would they have to be alive?

So, crude though the brain-part data were, they were all that were available for the functional and evolutionary questions we were asking.

Of course, the proof of the pudding is in the results!

Our new analyses showed that these relative data contained far more information than just size. The 'size' relationships from the species means alone were about 96% of the data; little else was left! Only 4% was about 'non-size' relationships. This is largely the same as the earlier simpler whole-brain, mean-size studies.

In contrast, the 'non-size' relationship in our new analyses was a huge 80%. They showed that all primates were separated from all insectivores, and both in turn from all bats, save for an 'origin' in our plots where the three groups intersected (Figure 8.5).

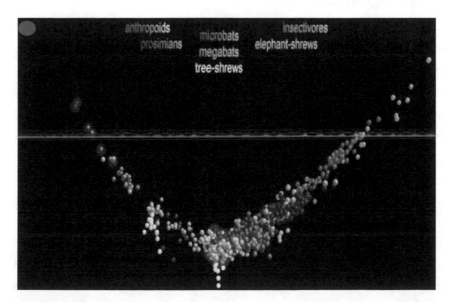

Figure 8.5: Analysis of relative brain part sizes in primates (reds and yellows on the left), in insectivores (greens on the right) and in bats (blues, lying centrally but actually projecting forward out of the plane of the others). The large red dot at the extreme top left is the human mean.

The whole result seems to be related to the major 'taxonomic' separations between primates, insectivores and bats! This is not surprising and, frankly, not all that interesting.

But, to our surprise, we also found arrangements between particular groups of species that seemed explicable only on the grounds of functional (behavioral) parallels.

For example, the fish-eating bats of the Old World fell with the fish-eating bats of the New World, rather than each with their own closer non-fish-eating bat relatives in each World. The main common feature seems to be very large feet for fish foraging.

Again, for example, the burrowing 'moles' of both New World and Old World insectivores fell together, rather than with each of their closer non-burrowing insectivore relatives on their own continents. The main common feature seems to be powerful upper limbs for burrowing.

Third, and of great interest to us, certain New World monkeys (the acrobatic woolly and spider monkeys) fell remarkably close to the Old World apes. This was even though these New World and Old World species are separated in evolutionary terms by many millions of years. The main common feature seems to be the specialized upper limb tree-climbing and tree-hanging behaviors of both.

We found many more such functional parallels among the other mammals.

Of course, these are bodily parallels. That is, we would expect to find parallels like these ***if we were looking at the bodies of these creatures***. Big feet are useful for fishing in fish-eating bats, whatever their hereditary relationships, and powerful upper

limbs are important in burrowing animals, whatever their evolutionary separations. Likewise, long arms might have evolved independently for arboreal activities in acrobatic apes and acrobatic
New World monkeys, whatever their genetic heritage. All are classical evolutionary parallels!

But we were not looking at their bodies; **we were looking at
their brains!**

In other words, we had found fascinating parallels in internal brain organization (at the crude, large-brain-part level).
Could such relationships among brain parts be related to bodily
behaviors?

But most workers, perhaps blinded by the original 96% relationship with overall size, felt that the different brains must be
only the result of a common or fundamental pattern of growth. It
is true that there is a common pattern of brain growth, but it would
seem unlikely for this to be the sole cause of these results!

> *Apparently challenging this idea:* **one basic pattern of**
> **growth** *was a major brain heresy.*
>
> But there was more to come.

The Brain Heresy Again: The Special Position of Humans!

Humans were separated by some 8 standard deviation units (the
measure provided by our particular form of analysis) from the
apes (first frame of Figure 8.6). This is likely mostly related to
the larger brains of humans over apes. However, we also found
that humans were separated from all primates (including apes) by
a further 22 units along higher statistical axes! In other words, we
had found a level of brain organization in humans (at this crude,

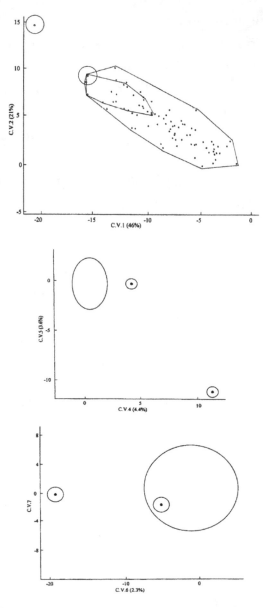

Figure 8.6:   The first frame shows the 8 standard deviation units of difference in axes one and two of humans (top left small circle) from all other primates. But the next two frames show further axes of the analysis (axes 4, 5, 6 and 7) in which humans alone, the distant small circle, are widely divergent from all other primates (large circle) and chimpanzees (the other small circle).

large-brain-part level) that does not exist in chimpanzees or any other primate (also Figure 8.6).

What part of the data produced this separation of humans? (Figure 8.7)

In other words, there is a level of brain organization in humans (at this crude, large-brain-part level) not found in chimpanzees, or indeed in any other nonhuman primate. The question is: what

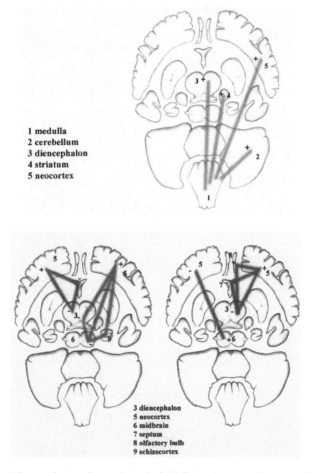

Figure 8.7: The top frame shows those links (all simple pairs) between the brain parts that contribute most to the size separations of all primates. But the two lower frames show those links, mostly triple and quadruple links, by which humans alone were separated from all primates (including apes) by a further 22 units along higher statistical axes!

produces this special human separation? It is not due to what separates all other primates.

It was clearly due to relationships among the major midbrain and forebrain parts alone. Further, many of these relationships involve links among three, four or even five particular brain parts; quite different from the simpler pairwise links in the all-primate separations. Given the enormous cognitive and behavioral differences between humans and nonhumans, this seems entirely reasonable.

Yet almost everyone else who has looked at brain sizes, blinded perhaps by the 96% relationship with body size and the 96% DNA similarity of humans and chimpanzees, has seen humans as just another ape. Indeed, we have been called 'the third chimpanzee'.

This finding, the idea of a marked human difference,
was the second heresy.

Most molecular factors place chimpanzees close to humans (Figure 8.8, upper frame). But molecular factors for the brain

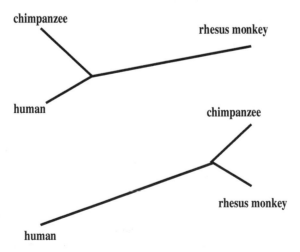

Figure 8.8:   Above: distance relationship between molecular factors for the liver, kidney, blood and bone. Below: distance relationships between molecular factors for the brain!

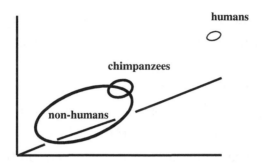

Figure 8.9:   The three-dimensional picture for plots of brain-part ratios uniquely separates humans from all other primates. The scale of this diagram is such that the separation of humans from other primates, when all statistical axes are included, is some 22 standard deviation units!

show that chimpanzees are closer to rhesus monkeys (Figure 8.8, lower frame).

Of these two molecular pictures, it is the second — the brain relationship — to which our brain-part-ratio data (as revealed by multivariate statistical methods) are most closely aligned (Figure 8.9).

The Brain Heresy a Third Time: Are We Still Evolving?

The very large difference between human and chimpanzee brains, and the newly increased time estimated since their separation, leads to another question. Could it be that in humans, changes in brain organization are partly due to a new form of evolutionary change? It would need to be one that implies very fast brain change, great elaboration of brain function/behavior, and both with totally new lifestyle possibilities.

The new changes in brain organization could stem in part from mechanisms for forming new connections not available to other species. Increased levels of brain inputs and outputs increase the number of dendrites and synapses within the rat brain — this kind of change is available in all species. But special effects in humans, caused by us ourselves (see later) and not possible to any but very minor degrees in other species, could have affected the human brain.

Thus, the level of external effects in developing humans is enormously greater than those in other species. For example, a singing, talking and touching (i.e., belly-caressing) pregnant woman and her partner can have influences upon their fetus and then, later, their baby, as evidenced by changed patterns of movement of the late fetus to sensations like sound and touch (and even sight — the fetus can 'see'), and of the early baby to seeing, singing, speaking and caressing. Likewise, the influences of siblings, grandparents and others close in the family may also have similar, if lesser, effects. These cannot easily occur, or occur to much lesser degrees, in most other species, even the great apes.

Such influences in humans, beginning in pregnancy, extended to infants, children and even teenagers, are therefore 'education' of a type. This covers not just formal education as we generally recognize it, but 'education' that stems from all influences, even in a fetus and infant that, despite being unable to speak, can yet vocalize and certainly see, hear, feel and communicate in their own way. Of course, in nonhuman primates, these initial influences presumably also exist, but they do not transpose into more complex, generation-crossing forms as they do with the continuity of human 'education'.

Brain organization comes through input/output effects on neuron development. Such effects not only modify the instructions of direct genetic factors, but also, through upstream and downstream factors, actually change the genetic instructions themselves. Ideas such as these were proposed theoretically by Waddington (the epigenetic landscape), by Moore (*The Dependent Gene*) and by Ridley (*Nature Via Nurture*). Such changes may even relate to the new findings by Fields about the functions of neuroglia, or special connective brain cells, and their development. These cells are far more numerous in human brains than that of other primates.

It is even not impossible that the soil for such change lies in the removal of constraints against improved brain structure and increased brain function provided by the relatively new evolution in humans of omnivory and the removal, therefore, of the brain-limiting effects in a higher primate of reduced animal protein and reduced vitamin B^{12}.

Waddington's metaphor helps give clarity, so let's put these concepts into pictures. He described development from the zygote to the adult as the path that a ball takes to roll down a hill (Figure 8.10). The original position of the ball near the top of the hill represents the (genetic) beginning. As the ball rolls down the hill, it describes the (epigenetic) pathway of development and growth. This pathway depends upon both the starting position (beginning genetic information) and the contours of the hillside (the various downstream epigenetic and environmental factors, as Waddington called them). The final position of the ball at the bottom of the hill represents adult form and function.

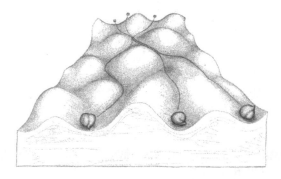

Figure 8.10: Waddington's epigenetic landscape from a starting gene, down the epigenetic landscape, to an adult.

With Waddington's metaphor in mind, let us examine the concept of a population. Figure 8.11 shows the situation where there is a population of genes. It diagrams how small starting positions of the ball (small population differences in genes) and gradually increasing changes in the landscape (increasing changes in the epigenetic factors) can produce large differences in the final position of the balls (differences among the population of adults). This alone does not imply any fundamental difference between humans and other forms.

Let us now include the effect of changes in the developmental landscape that are due to those changes in the contours *that are added by the organism (humans) because it can* (Figure 8.12).

Finally, however, we can envisage a situation where a generation can be changed by altering the landscape through the introduction of timing changes (i.e., earlier and earlier).

Thus Figure 8.13 shows how the change in the first frame of Figure 8.13 can be increased by the efforts of the still-living prior generations or materials from prior generations acting earlier and earlier in development.

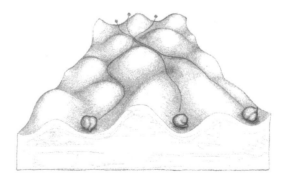

Figure 8.11:   Waddington's epigenetic pathway showing how slightly different zygotes may produce vastly different adults.

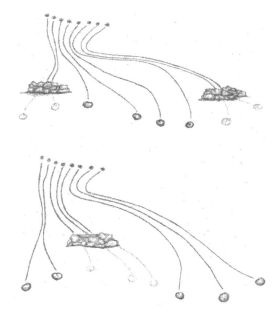

Figure 8.12: Upper frame: reducing variation by two changes in the contours, thus limiting the individuals as one close knit group. Lower frame: separating the species into two separate groups by introducing a different change in the contours. This seems to be standard.

This would be a form of change effected *by a population on its progeny because it can, and over time through education, in the wide sense*.

Such changes (Figure 8.13) could include: (a) the (now standard) effects of interactions between the various internal upstream and downstream molecular factors and the genetic factors themselves. But they could also include: (b) the effects of education from the new information technology mechanisms restricted to humans. They could include: (c) the complexity-increasing effects of a much greater volume of glia (if that concept is eventually proven); and:

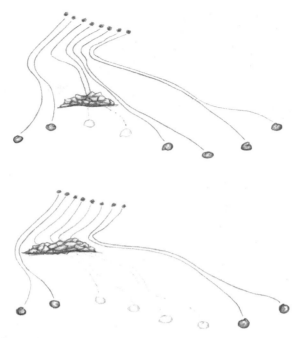

Figure 8.13:   Upper frame: increasing variation by late epigenetic effects eliminating some central individuals. Lower frame: greatly increasing variation by early epigenetic effects eliminating more central individuals (effects started earlier in lifetimes).

(d) the removal of animal protein-deficiency and cyanocobala-min-constraining limitations, but perhaps most of all (e) the various interactions that may occur between all these different influencing modalities. Figure 8.13 implies that the effect of all these factors might not only produce new forms for some adults

but also eliminate some adults that would
otherwise have been produced.

Of course, the genomes remain the same and so one would not expect this to produce evolution in the direct sense. However, it could result in a well-known situation that might nevertheless engender evolutionary change, which is that such a system might give rise to reproductive isolation that can greatly speed evolutionary separations. Given the normal breeding propensities of humans, this would seem, on the face of it, to be unlikely. However, let us go further.

This is the reverse of some prevailing theories and practices today, such as formal education starting later and later, often not until the ages of 6 or even 7 in parts of the USA. But it fits with educational systems of the past. For instance, education in Scotland started as early as 3–4 years old in my childhood. The Scottish teacher in my day would have been alarmed if her first task was to teach the child to read; it was expected that the child learnt to read at its mother's knee, while the teacher's first job was to teach the child to write and figure! Even so, the ordinary forms of education with which we are all familiar are unlikely to produce much sexual isolation in this way.

But a new form of education (hinted at above) that just might do this is the use of the computer and information technology, applied from increasingly younger ages, to increasingly limited portions of the population. Who amongst us has not been embarrassed by the 'teen, even the child, almost the infant, who knows how to 'work the machine' and is scathing that nanny and grandad can't? It is just possible that information technology may be doing something very interesting to the brains of information generations of humans. Would it be that we could cut up a few infants' brains to find out? Of course not! But the new non-invasive imaging methods might tell us something.

Of course, this might be strongly negative. We already hear voices warning about the dangers of computers to the very young. Uncontrolled access to computers and related gadgets by young children might well be strongly deleterious. *Homo nerdensis* might be an evolutionary liability!

Other changes, however, might be extremely powerfully positive, resulting in *Homo sapientior* (thanks to colleague Alan Harvey). I doubt that *Homo nerdensis* would very often breed with non-*nerdensis* forms; *nerdensis* seems so often to suffer from such major behavioral problems in getting on with its peers that breeding *in toto* might well be reduced or might even not occur (tongue in cheek here). But *Homo sapientior* may well seek out only its own! Already improvements in women's education seem to be associated with women tending to seek out only men who are educated at their own level or above. Are 'lesser' males being removed from the breeding pool of these 'super women'?

Are there really a number of new possibilities for the evolution of the human brain? Was Aldous Huxley (1946) correct in imagining his Alpha-intellectuals (given extra stimulation) and Delta-minuses (today's progeny of the drinking pregnant mum)? Was Julian Huxley (1957) correct in envisioning a new taxonomic group, the Psychozoa, containing at this point only humans? Was H. G. Wells (both himself, 1895, and his alter ego, David Lake, 1981) percipient in seeing Eloi and Morlocks in our human future?

Could *Homo* split (tongue in cheek)? Wow, what a heresy!

The Final Brain Heresy: Problems With Publishing!

A final brain heresy occurred as we tried to publish our first work. *Nature* turned the manuscript down 'in house' (i.e., not externally refereed). This is not unusual because *Nature* is flooded with great numbers of articles; many of them are very good, so not all can be taken! One accepts this kind of rebuff gracefully. It has happened to me many times!

However, not too long after that rejection, another paper appeared in *Nature* based on the means of the species (the published and therefore freely available, data of Stephan). This paper had carried out a somewhat similar study as our first. While it had not identified the enormous separation of humans (at that stage we had not emphasized that finding in our submission), it had recognized some of the ideas in our rejected manuscript.

How had that paper been published when our own far more sophisticated analysis on both species and individual statistics was rejected?

I thought about this and persuaded Willem that we should have a another try at *Nature*. We submitted what we thought was an improved paper and especially referred to the new *Nature* paper that was published since our first try. Again, two new versions of this were also turned down 'in house'!

I thought further about this, and after taking soundings from some neurobiological colleagues (remember, I am not, myself, a neurobiologist!), I decided to write personally to the editor of *Nature* about the decision. This is a correspondence that *Nature* generally doesn't enter into. It was certainly something that I would not lightly do, and I was very, very polite. But perhaps the editor realized that I had 'smelt a rat'.

We were, therefore, surprised but enormously pleased to be invited to present a yet further revision, which we did.

And this version **Nature** *published!*

Now I have had some 10 or so papers in *Nature* over the years (this is not boasting; 10 papers are not actually many when seen in the light of, at that point, a 50-year career). But it must be unusual for *Nature* to publish after three turn-downs!

And Now for Something Completely Different: The Hobbit Heresy!

Bones found at Liang Bua on the island of Flores in Indonesia, though thought to be at that time only 18,000 or so years old, were immediately and formally assessed as a new species, *Homo floresiensis*, perhaps a descendant of *Homo erectus*, perhaps an ancestor of local *Homo sapiens*, or even, as a few suggested, not *Homo* at all, but a nonhuman species perhaps similar to the australopithecines (notwithstanding that these latter are African and enormously older!).

Everyone was most excited when the finds were first announced. At the time, I was on a research trip to the USA, the UK and Europe. In the USA, I was given the chance to handle a computer-generated cast of the Liang Bua find, courtesy of Ralph Holloway at Columbia University. It happened while we were both at the annual meeting of the American Physical Anthropologists.

"Come to my hotel room,"
Ralph said, showing me the cast,
"and tell me what you think of this."

And later on, that same trip, I was able to spend an hour looking, albeit only through the glass cabinet, at the cast in the Science Museum, South Kensington.

Almost everyone had already decided that this skull was likely a new species. My first tentative observations agreed! I can document that I was in agreement because, when I returned from that trip, I immediately wrote a minute of my observations and tentative opinion that "it might be a new species that seemed to have primitive features." I circulated this document to our research students; they were all agog.

Some little time later, Peter Obendorf of the Royal Melbourne Institute of Technology asked me if I thought that these remains might be those of a cretin, probably a human cretin, though a cretin of some other species was also a possibility.

"Highly unlikely,"
I said to Peter without thinking. But then I started to think, remembering all my medical interests in bone and skeletons, growth and dwarfisms, and I decided that my negative opinion might have been precipitous.

Thus, this story starts with the concept of hypothesis testing: testing the idea of a new species. Here, testing means looking for evidence inconsistent with the hypothesis.

At first, of course, the tests were only tentative. I had not seen the materials (in fact, even now, neither Peter nor I have ever seen the materials, only casts and photographs), so our first studies depended on assessing the original published descriptions with photographs and measurements.

Various workers put forward several different hypotheses running along evolutionary, developmental and medical lines. The **evolutionary** idea was 'island dwarfing', the **developmental** idea was microcephaly (many different types exist) and the **medical** idea was Laron syndrome (rare overall, but present in 'carrier' populations).

Peter's suggestion was not evolution, development or disease, but environment (indeed, he is an environmental biologist). Small individuals (cretins) result from iodine-deficient mothers (Figure 8.14).

When Peter asked me what I thought about his cretinism idea, he did not know that he was asking someone who was especially attuned to that medical possibility. This is because I had had my medical education a long time ago. So long ago, indeed, that cretinism was still in the medical student curriculum. With my interests in bone, I had read about cretinism.

Not that cretinism still occurred in England when I was a medical student. No, preventative treatment had long been instituted.

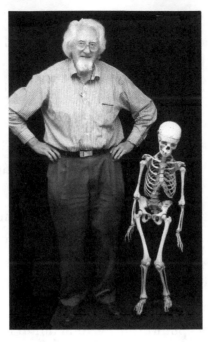

Figure 8.14:   Charles Oxnard and an adult (32-year-old) cretin; please do not mistake one for the other. Note the *unfused breast-bone segments in the adult cretin*, normally all fused in a 32-year-old human, but *normally unfused in a human child* (and *normally unfused in all adult apes!*).

After about 1900, no more cretins should have been born. But of course, cretins sometimes live to be 70 or 80, so some cretins were alive when I was a student, and thus it was still in the curriculum.

Therefore, when I thought more about Peter's suggestion, even though I had first told him he was crazy, I thought again and realized it might be possible. *All this came on the back of my having already told our students that it likely was a new species.*

Peter and I examined this new possibility tentatively in a first paper. It had to be tentative because we had not seen the materials. We depended upon what was published, and that was largely descriptive. Later we were joined by Ben Kefford (then at the University of Technology, Sydney) for additional biological and statistical support.

Our combined view that it might be a cretin raised a furore. Some workers were quite impolite:

> *"I am very sorry indeed to see serious scientists involved in such a travesty."*

was one widely distributed comment! We were flayed through the media: paper, wireless, television and electronic. Everyone *knew* the new species idea was the last word. Our attempts at publication were stymied.

Indeed, one very prestigious journal put our manuscript through three separate sets of reviews (which was already slightly unusual). One referee, initially only somewhat doubtful, became increasingly and antagonistically opposed with each revision. The paper was turned down.

Another journal turned the manuscript down in just 24 hours because of the immediate report of one — just one — reviewer who simply said only that:

> *"Under no circumstances should this work be published!"*

Eventually, however, the *Proceedings of the Royal Society* took the paper (so they weren't all bad). Even here, one reviewer implied that the *PRS* only took the paper because 'Charles' was a Fellow! He got it wrong. Prince Charles was a Fellow, but Charles Oxnard certainly was not.

In the following years, more and more information appeared about 'the Hobbit', as this tiny adult had been quickly dubbed. There were good measurements and clear photographs. As a result, we could more properly compare it with cretins. This strengthened our ideas.

Thus, our title changed from a question in our 2008 paper on the skull: "Are the small human-like fossils found on Flores human endemic cretins?" to our statement in the 2010 paper: "Post-cranial skeletons of hypothyroid cretins show a similar anatomical mosaic as *Homo floresiensis.*"

Even with these more concrete data, we had great difficulty getting the idea published. Journal editors consistently sent it to protagonists for review, and it was as consistently rejected. It was only when one editor of one journal (*PLoS ONE*), after three separate sets of reviews and our responses to them, smelt a rat. He took a great chance and published it (2010)!

But our idea was still completely denied in 2012 in a short paper entitled '*Homo floresiensis* is not a modern human cretin'. The reasons for denial sound persuasive. They stated that we had never seen the Hobbit specimens; that there was no evidence in the Hobbit of slowed growth and development like the unfused epiphyses of cretins; that the limb proportions in the Hobbit were not as in cretins; that there were no bone torsions and angles in the Hobbit as in cretins; and last, that there was no evidence of iodine deficiency on Flores, the *sine qua non* for cretinism there.

Yet our 2010 paper (mentioned above) demonstrated exactly the existence of these cretin anatomical features in the Hobbit. Let us look just at unfused epiphyses; these are clearly evident in the Hobbit in the wrist, knee cap, fibula, a foot bone, a vertebra and a poorly figured sternum; an impressive array! In other parts where the Hobbit (if a cretin) might have shown unfused epiphyses, the epiphyses (in their original papers described as 'absent') were now described as 'damaged'.

However, the last contention that the Hobbit could not have been a cretin "because there is no iodine deficiency in Flores" was in a different ballpark.

In fact, we had reported on surveys documenting severe iodine deficiency on Flores. In 1996, there were 41% of visible goiters, and in 2003, 51%. An Indonesian medical report in 2008 recorded that there was "severe endemic iodine deficiency in 31% of primary school children ... [and] ... in 43.4% of pregnant women in Flores, with the most severely affected district ... [being] ... Manggarai" (Manggarai is the locality where the Hobbit was found). We have recently found 1970s photographs of many Manggarai women and many 1930s Indonesian village school children with visible goiters.

Of course, such findings imply that humans and other mammals living in Flores today should show cretinism, and they do. But they also imply that even extinct species might also show cretinism. Cretinism is no respecter of species or time!

The opposition also did not tackle our further (1910) questions. One was: why had the Hobbit bones not been dated? The dates given for the Hobbit at the time, circa 18,000 years, were based merely upon dating the site (and newer studies are suggesting that the site is very much older still)! But the date of a site is not necessarily the date of the bones. Dating of bones is now a totally routine and necessary test in archeology!

A second question, was: why were the Hobbit bones not examined for DNA? The bones were not fossil casts; they were soft, 'the consistency of wet blotting paper', when first found!

Actually, their DNA *has* been tested, several times, **but the results have never been published!** Is this because they show only modern human DNA, which is not consistent with the idea of a new species?

In fairness, a human-like DNA result could well be rejected as modern contamination. Modern DNA in the Hobbit could have come from the many Indonesian and Australian workers who have handled the bones. However, if that were so, then that human DNA would include both Australian and Indonesian DNA, and these could be distinguished. But if the DNA was only Indonesian, then there would be no reason why only Indonesian handlers, and not Australian, would be so involved. This would imply that the most likely situation would be if the Hobbit *were* an Indonesian — and very much human — cretin!

Therefore, I ask again: why have these DNA results not been reported, a totally necessary test in archeology?

> *This, then, is the most recent heresy (though I do feel others growing inside me!).*

Yet I am not indissolubly 'wedded' to these ideas. To be 'wedded' would imply that I had fallen into the same uncritical trap. **I will be more than happy to eat my words** if the idea can be tested to destruction.

Do These Three Heresies Have Futures?

So far, the first of these three heresies, the one about the australopithecines, has now turned out to be more right than wrong.

The second one about human brains seems, so far, at least equivocal. There is not enough certainty either way. Yet even now, in 2021, publications are starting to recognize our side of the matter.

The third, on the Hobbit, is generally still believed to be wrong. But perhaps not enough time has passed. Perhaps the DNA evidence will appear; then we may know what the hobbit really was!

> *Being a heretic is a very important part of doing research!*

9 Guessing Human Pasts, 'Guestimating' Human Futures

As already explained, my aim for medicine came from that Scottish schoolmaster who said:

"There are things called science we dinna teach in this skule. Here, ye'd better be reading these."

And he threw at me writings (in English) from Goethe, Wegener, Thompson and Zuckerman. As a result, even from the beginning, my interest in medicine was mixed up with an interest in evolution.

Goethe, about 400 years ago, had a fascinating idea (Goethe was an anatomist as well as a writer of Faust). It was that the human skull came from many spinal vertebrae compressed together. At age 9, I believed it — his picture of the skull seemed so reasonable. In 1952, during my first research at university, I was shocked to learn that it was not so.

The skull is segmented, just not like the backbone!

But it was nearly so; Goethe was almost right.

Wegener, 100 years ago, proposed that the continents had drifted apart. At age 9, I believed it. Again, his picture — of South America fitting into Africa — was so convincing that I never knew that everyone thought Wegener was nuts. So, in my first university year (1952), I could not understand:

why everyone was high on plate tectonics.

I had always known it was so from Wegener.

D'Arcy Thompson in 1917 used a pictorial idea, borrowed from Descartes, to describe differences in the anatomies of animals. At age 9, I was convinced,

> *again, entranced by pictures.*

In 1952, while at university, I started using Thompson's ideas.

Finally, Solly Zuckerman, in the 1930s, wrote a book called *Functional Affinities of Man* (sic), *Monkeys and Apes*. As a result, I decided I wanted to work with him (the only one of those authors still alive at that time). How silly for a school boy to think he could work with such a distinguished individual as Zuckerman, later confidant of Prime Ministers, friend of Monarchs!

> *Yet I did, from 1952, as a first-year student,*
> *and on and off til his death at 88.*

Dr. Watson, that Little Old Scottish School Master, could have had no idea of the lifetime effect he would have on that small boy. Why on earth, in 1942, did he not give me Darwin's ***On the Origin of Species***? Perhaps Scottish religion got in the way!

Years Pass, and I Come to Los Angeles

A hundred miles down the coast from Los Angeles is the Institute for Creation Science. They are delighted at my arrival. After all, isn't Oxnard the scientist who debunks Darwinism? Isn't he anti-evolution?

If you don't believe me, google my name. Several hundred hits are on my evolutionary research papers and books. Many thousands of hits are about the City of Oxnard in California (to be expected). But tens of thousands of hits are about how my studies, and those of Zuckerman, Ashton, and of our various students and colleagues, because they 'test' conventional stories of human evolution, provide support for Creation science! And there is nothing I can do about it. You try removing rubbish from the internet!

More Years Pass and I Arrive in Australia

Because the winning of research funds in the USA had gradually become harder and harder (until one's eventual 'take' was reduced to only one in every five or six applications), when I first arrived in Australia, I applied for 6 grants. I was almost embarrassed to get three! The golden age of research, dead in England and dying in the USA, was then still present in Australia. That was AD 1987: AD meaning Anti-Dawkins (John, not Richard!). For a further thirty years in Australia, external grant successes continued.

However, in contrast, my first internal research grant application at the University of Western Australia failed!

I applied again the next year. Failed!

And the year after that. Failed!

Then I appointed Nina Jablonski from abroad (in those days professors appointed academics). I tell her this story. She smiled, gently.

"Oh,"
she said,
"just delete the word 'evolution' from the title of your research proposals."

She had learnt this from the Women's Group on campus, an organization to which I did not have access. Next year proved her right. Success!

Also, when I came to Australia, I discovered that 43% of medical students in Melbourne believed in special creation. I have never dared ask this question of the medical student cohorts in Western Australia!

Thus, you can see: the mores of my Scottish Schoolmaster in the forties, and the US Creation Science Institute in the seventies, were still alive and well in UWA in the nineties. And to a degree, it is still so today: a 'legacy' of Darwin!

Darwin's Legacies

The above story, for me, is the 'unwanted legacy' of Darwin. In contrast, my 'wanted legacy' from Darwin stems from a quotation. I am sure we all have our favorites.

Darwin wrote:

"All living things have much in common, in their internal metabolic processes, their ultrastructural and molecular relationships, their intracellular organelles and intranuclear complexities, their genetic, developmental and reproductive patterns, and their immunological tolerances and resistances."

Of course, I lie.

Darwin's actual words were:

"All living things have much in common, in their chemical compositions, their cellular structures, their germinal vesicles, their laws of growth and reproduction, and their liabilities to injurious substances. And if we admit these, we must likewise admit that all the organic beings which have ever lived on this earth are descended from one primordial form."

Darwin's are the words, Darwin's is the book, changing forever the way we see evolution. Yet Darwin, through his *On the Origin of Species*, was very careful about human origins. Darwin only briefly recognized the similarities of humans and apes. He was well aware of the implications of his 'dangerous idea'!

Today, David Attenborough, for instance, documents this for the full sweep of life on earth. I here use the words to summarize it for humanity alone.

Ever since Darwin (a famous phrase), we anatomists have been dissecting away all those bits of the human body that are common to apes and humans.

The heart, the kidneys, the liver and the lungs can go — they are essentially the same in apes and humans (even, nowadays, occasionally interchangeable!).

Muscles and bones can go — they are essentially the same in apes and humans (except for a few little bits in apes: e.g., one small muscle in the arm enjoying the sonorous title of latissimo-dorso-condyloideus-epitrochlearis [I love long words!] and one small bone in the wrist, the os centrale). Yet the 'ghosts' of even these apparently unimportant ape structures exist in every human in unexpected ways!

Even the brain can go too — 96.6 percent of the brain in apes and humans is simply the result of body size!

Is nothing left? What about behavior, taxonomy, classification, relationship?

Ever since Darwin, behaviorists have been chipping away.

'Only Man' (sic) uses tools. No, lots of animals use tools.

Aha, only Man (sic) makes tools. No, a number of animals make tools, even some very surprising ones.

Aha, aha, only Man (sic) makes tools for future use. No, some animals do even this.

Does no behavior separate us and others?

Ever since Darwin, taxonomists have demoted *Homo* (Man, sic). We have been demoted from our zoological superfamily (named after us, the *Hominoidea*), down to our own family (the *Hominidae*), down again to our own subfamily (the *Homininae*), down, again, to our own species (*Homo sapiens*). We are even relegated by some all the way down to mere subspecies status, *Homo sapiens sapiens*, alongside some fossils (e.g., *Homo sapiens neanderthalensis*).

All the way down we have been trailed by apes. Some suggestions even include apes in *Homo*.

Are things starting to reverse?

The View After Darwin!

I have one distinguished colleague (Professor Alan Harvey) who suggested elevating *Homo sapiens* (Man [sic] the Wise) of yesterday's thirty thousand years ago to *Homo sapientior* (Man [sic] the Wiser) of tomorrow. Would this be a new subspecies, I wondered! And could the ghosts of yesteryear be pointing toward visions for the future?

Could modern humans actually split? I do not mean into the Morlocks and Eloi of Wells' *Time Machine*, but from *Homo sapientior* (above) into both *Homo sapientissimus* (Man [sic] the Wisest) and *Homo nerdensis* (Man [sic] the 'Nerd'). These last would be in a transition from the Fishing-Net and the Butterfly-Net to the InterNet and the TwitterNet! I will return to this theme later.

Thus, when I was a scientific child, I accepted, as a child of that day, that the common ancestor of modern humans and modern apes lived 20, 25 or even 30 million years ago.

This was a respectable degree of distance, one that the Bishop's wife could tolerate. As she said:

"I hear Mr. Darwin has said that we may be descended from an ape. I hope that it be not true. But if it be true, I pray that it become not widely known!"

But when I became a scientific man, I put away childish things. New ideas from fossil anatomies, animal behaviors, concepts of molecules and sizes of brains have all been drawing the human/ape relationship ever closer — eventually indecently close, at one point to less than 3 million years ago! The culmination of this trend is the oft-quoted DNA factoid that humans are 98.6% chimpanzees. Of course, we are also 96% orang utans, 90% rats, and even 55% bananas.

Now, in my scientific dotage, I perceive a re-reversal. New fossils and new molecules are pushing our common ancestry with the apes further back — back from that 3-million-year figure to 5 million years, 8 million years, 10 million years and, most recently, perhaps even back to more than 13 million years. Could it be that we actually are more different from the apes than we previously assumed?

Of course, not all of our parts are different from the apes! Human livers, kidneys, spleens, bloods, bones, etc, are all extremely similar to ape livers, kidneys, spleens, bloods, bones, etc. Together, they are all markedly different from monkey livers, kidneys, ... etc.

But, when it comes to brains, it is humans that are vastly different. Human brains are an incredible 20 times more different from ape and monkey brains than these latter are from each other.

And human brains seem to have been changing, especially recently, perhaps 10 times more quickly than ape and monkey brains (see previous chapter).

Implications for Humans?

Could this involve a form of evolution not available to animals, a form due to the interactions of genetic blueprints, developmental processes and environmental factors in a species that is capable of the changes that we, as humans, alone, can make in ourselves?

Such changes occur down the generations, along the families, across the communities, and among the tribes. They derive from guarding tradition, knowledge and history, through both teaching the old and discovery of the new. They involve, initially, the linking of pictures, symbols, music and rhythms, at first in temporary form (able to be passed between communicating individuals), and then more permanently (as the tablet, the book and the gramophone record are passed down the generations), and finally, electronically, by the computer, the eye-phone, information technology, and the cloud, all these spanning an entire world and all these for no other creature.

Modern Humans Among the Fossils: 'Guestimations'

Such thinking meant that I have long been dissatisfied with the current ways of assessing human evolution from studies of fossils. The relationships of fossils have been described in a variety of different ways (Figure 9.1).

The first three of these models are commonly used in cartoons of human origins (Figure 9.2).

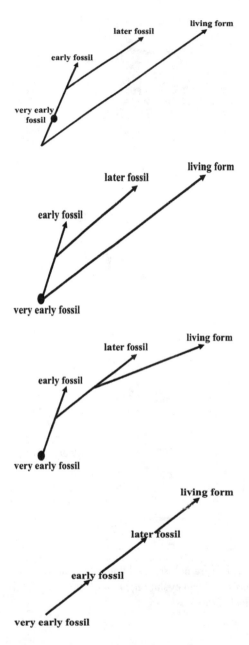

Figure 9.1: Four (among many) ways of describing relationships between fossils and the living.

Top frame: linear transmutations.
Second frame: branching changes.
Third frame: few fossils give rise to living forms.
Fourth frame: no found fossil gives rise to the living.

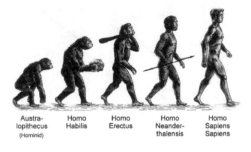

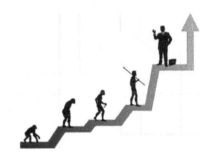

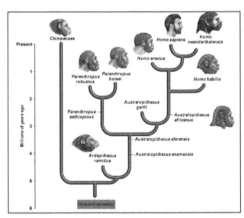

Figure 9.2:   Linear (first frame), stepped linear (second frame), and branching (third frame) 'guestimations' of human evolution, *in all of which most fossils are assumed to be direct or close relatives of humans!*

Of course, pictures like the above were first worked out by comparing the anatomical features of living species and fossils (the latter usually incomplete). Today they also arise from molecular (genetic) comparisons (again, of which the data for fossils are

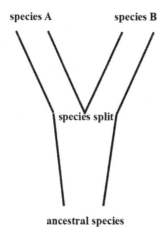

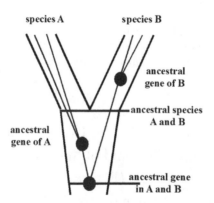

Figure 9.3:   The timing of ancestral species splits based on anatomies (above) is likely to be very different from the timing of splits based on ancestral genes (below).

usually very incomplete). But there can be problems. Figure 9.3 shows how molecules may give quite different answers than anatomies.

Thus, I was not happy with the standard views. But, though I knew that it might be possible to model such concepts computationally, my own computer skills were not good enough. So, I decided to simulate different possibilities by tossing dice to make 'evolutionary' decisions. This has been done before in science (even if Einstein famously said, "God does not play dice"). Of

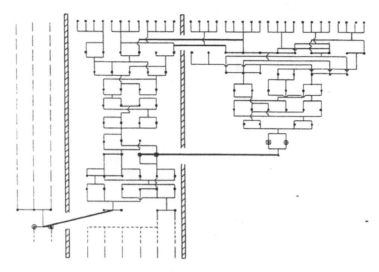

Figure 9.4:   A simple genealogy of individuals starting from a male/female pair from one region (bottom left in the diagram), migrating across a barrier (the left hatched vertical line) to a second region already containing individuals, and then producing its own descendants.

course, the game was very simple. I tried to imitate the effects, on genealogies, of 'breeding' and of 'migrations'. At first, I did it simply with male/female pairs (Figure 9.4).

In this model, particular descendants then migrated again (twice) to a third region, one fairly soon after the first migration, and one later. Next, I converted this diagram to show only the links from the first migration (Figure 9.5).

But one migration leading to a link with other individuals gives rise to more migrations, creating a more complex picture (Figure 9.6).

I then tried slightly more complex modelling, this time of species rather than individuals (Figure 9.7).

Drawing inferences from the found-fossil species alone almost always leads to totally false relationships. For example, the left-hand analysis of Figure 9.7 implies that all the living forms

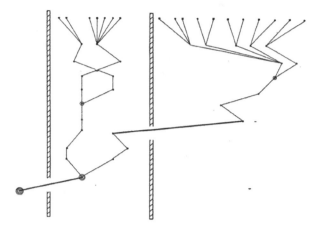

Figure 9.5:   The effect of the migration suggests a complete separation between the groups across the barriers (simulated migrations).

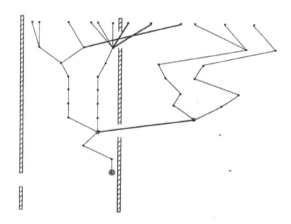

Figure 9.6:   Further migrations indicate that different individuals led to other migrations.

arose from a single, very recent fossil. The right-hand analysis (the correct analysis) shows that the extant species actually separated very much further back in time.

These models might have gone no further (though they have been accepted and published), had I not met Dr. Ken Wessen. Ken Wessen, already with a PhD in theoretical plasma physics,

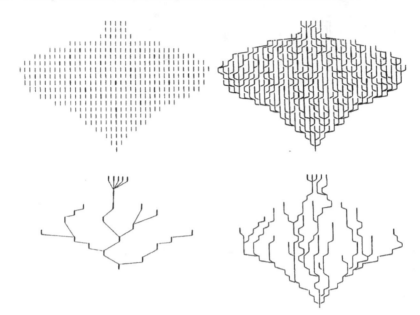

Figure 9.7: A computer-simulated genealogy of species (the small vertical lines), starting with an initial species and evolving into an ampulla-shaped pattern of species.

The upper left-hand frame shows all species, both found species (i.e., fossils, bold vertical lines) and not-found species (light vertical lines).

The lower left-hand frame shows the paleontologist's view from found-fossil species alone. The upper right-hand frame shows the true relationships among all the species. The lower right-hand frame shows the true relationships of the found-fossil species alone. This last, the true picture, is completely different from the paleontologist's assessment (lower left-hand frame).

did a doctoral degree with me applying his computational skills in mathematical modelling to evolutionary biology. His PhD thesis was the shortest I have ever supervised — 213 pages as published by Cambridge University Press — and he received honors for it. (Another student, Dr. Vanessa Hayes, wrote the longest thesis I have ever supervised: three very fat volumes, 467 pages; it is also a superb thesis with an enormous body of data!)

Ken set up species-divergence and population-genealogy modelling systems.

Ken Wessen's Species-Divergence System for Modelling Evolution

The first of these systems allowed for changes in:
numbers of species generations,
numbers of characters for each species,
numbers of states for each character,
rate of change of characters,
selective advantages of characters, and
possibility of divergence or merging (simulating speciation and hybridization).

Figure 9.8 shows how species lineages in such models might change from an initial species (at the base of the diagrams) to present-day species (top of the diagrams). Found-fossil species are indicated as solid circles, the non-found species by open circles. Lineages are shown by lines.

Another effect is shown in Figure 9.9. The various factors have, in this case, allowed the pattern of evolution of species (upper left frame) to give rise to a species structure with a narrow neck (as due, for example, to climactic, geologic and astronomic factors, amongst others).

Another example (Figure 9.10) isolates the implications of migrations and shows, *in toto*, that the information about the fossils alone may (as in this example) not allow correct identification of any migrations.

The implications of doing many such runs are shown in Table 9.1. The true common ancestors are always much further back in time than the common ancestors calculated from the fossils alone.

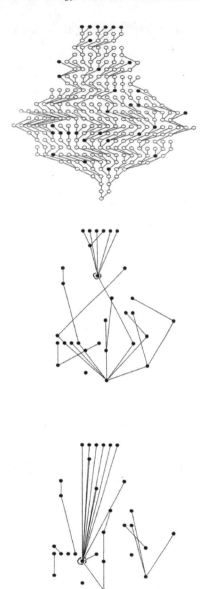

Figure 9.8: Top shows the complete model (top frame) with fossils shown in bold. Middle shows the relationships calculated from fossils alone. Bottom shows that this is spurious; the real common ancestor is far back in time!

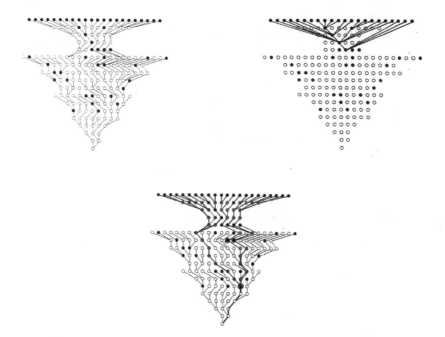

Figure 9.9: The upper left frame shows all species, found-fossil species (dark), un-found species (clear) and the links between them. The upper right frame shows the relationships of present-day species as calculated by the paleontologist from the known fossils. The ancestor of all the extant species is only 5 species generations back in time. The lower frame shows the real ancestors of the living species at the top. Three quite different lineages are apparent. The true ancestral species of all the extant species is far back in time, only 6 species-generations from the base of the model.

A final example (Figure 9.11) indicates the complexities of both migrations and splits.

The species lineages have completely different evolutionary pathways and completely different earliest ancestors in their migrations (Figure 9.12).

Of course, one has to make many runs of models like these to get the statistics (Table 9.2). For example, the true numbers (averages) of fossil species lying on lineages leading to modern forms are many less than the apparent numbers. Moreover, the

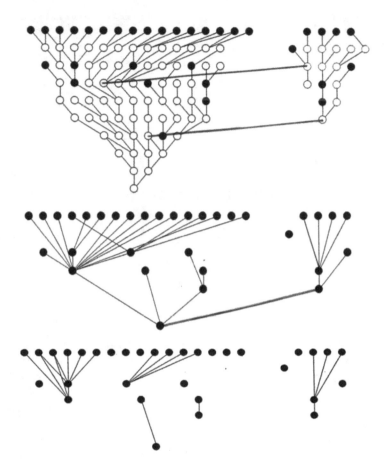

Figure 9.10:   The upper frame shows the real (modelled) effects of migrations with the true migrations being indicated as bold lines. The middle frame shows the migration (bold) that seems evident through looking only at modelled data for the fossils. An incorrect migration is indicated! The lowest frame shows that no fossils are involved in the migrations at all.

'real' common ancestor of all the living species is far older (much further down) than the (wrongly) 'assumed' ancestor.

Most fossils are likely not on any lineages leading to today's species,
and yet today's paleoanthropologists place most fossils on lineages
leading to the present day!

Table 9.1: Differences between apparent and true fossil links.

Number of runs	Generations back to true common ancestor	Generations back to apparent common ancestor
52	18 (range 15–23)	8 (range 3–11)
28	0	10 (range 6–16)
20	0	0

Number of runs	True number of fossils on lineages leading to extant species	Apparent number of fossils on lineages leading to extant species
1,000	11 out of 34	25 out of 34

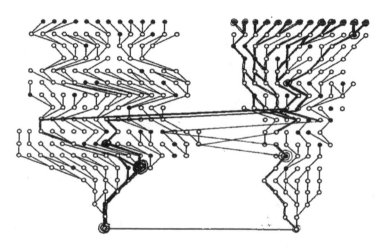

Figure 9.11: Again, solid dots are 'fossil' species (therefore known). Open dots are species that existed, but were not 'fossilized'. Because we know all the links, we are able to draw lines connecting both found and unfound species. The different bold lines follow the different relationships. Circled species show first ancestors for each lineage.

Ken Wessen's Population-Genealogy System for Modelling Breeding

Ken's next system included: varieties of mating patterns, fertility chances, consanguineous mating, infidelity factors, adding genetics to the modelling, varying mutation rates, genetic recombination rates, and, again, migration possibilities and selection factors, and

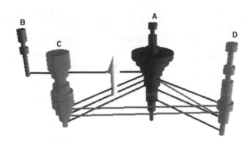

Figure 9.12:   An example of migrations among four 'continents' and over many species generations (details hidden by the many generations, but present in the numerical output).

Table 9.2:   Number of fossils lying on extinct lineages.

Number of runs	True average number of fossils lying on lineages leading to present-day species	Apparent average number of fossils reconstructed as lying on lineages leading to present-day species
1,000	14 out of 34	22 out of 34

yet again, other features, such as individual genealogies (reproduction) and molecular 'changes' (genetics). Using this, could we model the effects, over hundreds of generations, and of different numbers and mortality of offspring? Could the numbers of offspring affect the positions of ancestors (e.g., ancestral mothers, ancestral fathers)? Figure 9:13 shows three runs.

We then wondered if we could model the effects of different mating patterns, such as monogamy, polygyny and polyandry (Figure 9.14 and Table 9.3).

Third, we examined the effects of a 'one-child policy' (Figure 9.15). This single example suggested that the ancestral parents were located about midway through the generations.

But, of course, this was just one single run. Many runs yielded pictures like the following (Figure 9.16).

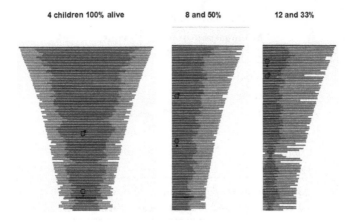

Figure 9:13: The first frame shows the generations produced over time (upwards in the diagram) from the initial seeding. Following back down from the top (present day), it finds the first male (father) and female (mother) of all living people (when using an average of 4 children per breeding pair and all live). The second and third frames (showing only half models, because they are symmetrical about the midline) have 8 children on average (but half die) and 12 children on average (but two-thirds die). The average overall number of children is the same, but the effects of modelled birth and death rates, of course, determine completely different first parents!

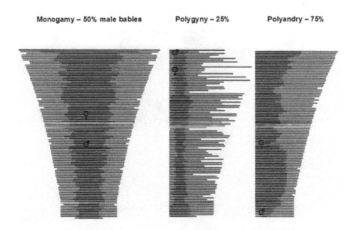

Figure 9.14: The differences in lineages in the three different mating systems. The polygyny and polyandry simulations show only half plots (symmetrical around the midline). The male and female icons show that the first mothers and fathers are in completely different generations in the different systems. Table 3 shows a sample of such statistics from many runs.

Table 9.3:   Mating patterns.

**Monogamous model: 10 runs,
25 generations, 3 continents.**

using random samples	common ancestors
female average	12th generation
male average	16th generation
using entire population	common ancestors
female average	6th generation
male average	14th generation

**Polygynous model: 10 runs, 25 generations,
3 continents, and it went extinct three times.**

using random samples	common ancestors
female average	16th generation
male average	9th generation
using entire population	common ancestors
female average	13th generation
male average	7th generation

One child on average

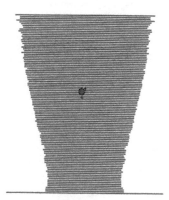

Figure 9.15:   One run of a one-child policy.

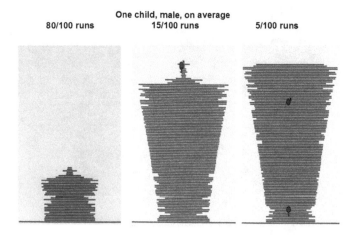

Figure 9.16:   The effects, over 100 generations, of one-child policies!

Most of the time (80%), as one would expect, the entire population dies out. Fifteen times the population just makes it to the present day. Only 5 times does the population survive well.

Finally, we moved from effects involving reproduction (of individuals, babies and mating pattern, as above) to effects at the level of individual chromosomes (Figure 9.17).

All this implies that the real picture of human evolution is more complicated, allows for a greater range of possibilities and, despite much more data, or in fact ***perhaps because of much more data***, is now ***much more tentative*** than has ever been recognized before.

Single certainty is, ***at last***, giving place to **many tentative possibilities!** This idea is especially illuminating in the latest stages of human evolution.

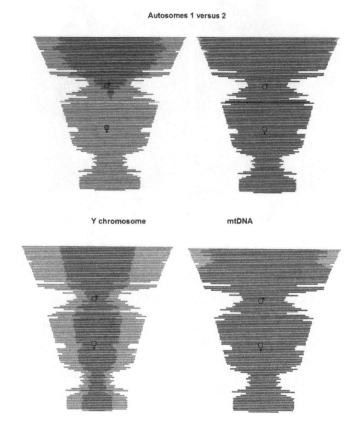

Figure 9.17:   Different effects of studying autosomes (above) and sex chromosomes (below). (So far, more models to give statistics have not been carried out.)

Resultant New Thinking About Human Evolution

Many fossils believed to be related to humans have now been named, from *Sahelanthropus* and *Orrorin* perhaps 8 to 6 million years ago, through *Ardipithecus* at say 6 to 4 million years ago, through various *Australopithecines* at say 4 to 2 million years ago, to twelve (at last count) species of fossil *Homo* (*including erectus, neanderthalensis but not sapiens!*) at say 2 million years ago and less, and then through ancient *sapiens* species on to the present. Although the precise evolutionary assessments of relationship among these different named groups differ somewhat among different workers, depending upon precisely how the fossils are assessed, they are almost all thought to lead (almost inexorably, one might say) to modern humans.

Only those fossils representing various forms of robust *Australopithecus* (originally also believed to be human ancestors) are usually now placed on sidelines at around 4 to 2 million years. However, even these are still, by most workers, believed to be closely related, being only slightly offset from the main line leading to modern humans.

It is surprising that there are no fossils judged
as related to modern apes!

It is even more surprising that there are no fossils
unrelated to apes or humans!

It is most surprising of all that almost everything
'belongs to the human part of the tree'!

Of course, the modelling studies carried out here can't tell us what did happen. But they do imply, most strongly, that we should expect:

most lines leading only to extinct dead ends,
many lines rejoining to form new hybrids and subspecies, and
many lines of migrations within regions, across mainlands and between continents.

This is contrary to conventional wisdom, but starting to be supported by new studies.

First, today's paleontological investigations see so many more fossils that it is highly likely that they lie in complex spreading 'bushes' or in complicated interacting 'reticulations' rather than in a few simple 'branches', and certainly not in single 'twigs'.

Second, today's biomechanical studies of the anatomies are suggesting more complex functional and behavioral possibilities.

Third, today's ecological studies negate the simple idea that human evolution occurred on relatively treeless plains, eschewing most other environmental possibilities.

Fourth, today's modelling studies imply that migrations have been very numerous and very complex, negating the idea of a very few major migrations.

Fifth, and most importantly, today's molecular data—obtained sometimes from fossils and especially from living forms — imply complicated genetic interrelationships.

Thus, it is not surprising that the models above suggest greater evolutionary complexity.

Notwithstanding all this, the temptation of fossil hunters and storytellers is still to see almost every new find as especially important! The number of fossils that, when first found, are immediately designated as 'critical' or the 'earliest' or the 'most important', or 'pre-human' or even 'human', still seems unusually large. The number that might be ancestors of apes is still incredibly small (at present, one fossil pre-chimpanzee only, and with just a few teeth). The number that just might be neither ancestral to apes nor to humans seems to be almost zero!

Human Evolution: From There to Here, and Further

The next question relates to humans today. The 7 billion people who inhabit the earth all belong to one species of human which we label *'Homo sapiens'*, which in English means 'wise man', or better, 'rational human' in today's vernacular.

But many people believe that 'humans' comprise large numbers of separate 'races', 'ethnicities' or 'tribes', or belong to 'specific language groups', 'specific lands' or 'specific religions', and so on: all very separate!

Of course, most other mammal species comprise much smaller populations living in far more restricted areas and with far fewer chances of widespread reproductive or other contacts. For example, the monkey species in Sulawesi, a somewhat star-shaped island, comprise a small number of separately recognizable subspecies along the 'arms of the star', where agonistic interactions sometimes occur and where local hybrids, usually infertile, also exist in small intermediate zones (Gene Albrecht's thesis, and other papers).

In contrast, the 7 billion humans today are all, in general, interbreedable. At earlier times, fossil groups (I say groups, but usually these finds may consist of as little as a single bone) that we now call Denisovans, Neanderthalers, Erectus and Luzonians (and almost certainly many more that have not yet been found, or if found, have not yet been named) were not like those monkey hybrids on Sulawesi. They differed from them in their gradually increasing numbers, in moving across and into land areas of others. Such migrations could include not only the travels of groups looking for good lands or leaving bad lands, but also the movements of 'travelling salesmen', the invasions of armies (with camp followers) and the returns of battle winners (with captives) which, as a result, bring about *complex interchanges of genes over many thousands — indeed hundreds of thousands — of years.*

As a result, it is not surprising that humans today, despite so often self-identifying as separate groups with different skin colors, special languages, particular social and cultural relationships, recognitions of family links (often spurious), individual agonistic activities, specific group aggressions, even separate religions and land areas, are not really separate. We are a 'pan-species'.

We share genes very widely among ourselves. I myself have Asian genes, even though there is no record of this in my family history! (If there were, the knowledge might have been suppressed). Further, however, humans today also contain genes from the fossil individuals of yesteryear. A quite large 2 percent to as much as 8 percent of our genomes today contains genes from these older fossil groups. Thus, genes from early humans can be found in all of today's modern humans, whether from Africa, Eurasia, the Americas, or even Australia. And the story is not by any means complete — genes from four other ancient human groups, currently unidentified, are also known in Southeast Asia and Africa! Even in indigenous Australia, genes of Neanderthals and Denisovans occur, together with at least one other unidentified group.

Given all this human admixture, why do so many of us persist in seeing 'sharp human racial' separations?

These separations started for me in the (artificial) distinction between Town and Gown in Old Britain. They are evident in many other artificial ways: from upstream to downstream water rights, across land rights and sea rights, from landowners to renters to squatters, between rich and poor, across left and right parties, among democratic and autocratic nations, among the strictly held religions, and through the antagonisms of tribes, warring factions, genocidal maniacs, and so on! And all this seems to have become especially hardened at the present time.

Why do we persist in accepting such sharp human separations, such races? Why indeed?

Many of these thoughts are just like the few small pebbles with which I have played on Newton's beach. They are the musings of a single not very well-known, not especially brilliant, and certainly never very highly cited investigator.

But even these few pebbles have the capacity to make me wonder about the way human evolution is described by our discipline, how it is introduced by teachers of all kinds to students, how it is largely presented by the media and perceived by the general public, and how it bolsters the degree of present day social and political separations. Do we need to think again about all this?

10 Chapter

Gold Standards, Accepted Wisdoms, Best Practices: Are they Crippling Straitjackets?

'Gold standards', 'accepted wisdoms' and 'best practices' are often said to be what we should strive for in research, as in life. They sound good. Can they, however, be 'straitjackets', the very restraints that stop us going further?

First: 'Gold Standards' and Spongy Bone

Studies of the external shapes of bones by observation and measurement described earlier, naturally led on to studies of the interior of bones: characterizing internal patterns. While external shape can be measured, at its simplest with a ruler, internal pattern seemed a more difficult problem. In those days, the internal structure could only be examined by cutting sections or taking radiographs. They showed that the interior of a bone has complex patterns and textures that are not easily 'measured'.

However, the day arrived (a story told elsewhere in this book) where it seemed that, rather than trying to measure many individual elements of a pattern, one might try to characterize the whole pattern, or the whole texture, in an overall manner. I had set this problem on one side.

But today, bone patterns and textures can be studied in many different and sophisticated ways due to the enormous growth of computer power, imaging modes and mathematical complexity.

I was drawn first to the use of Fourier transforms by seeing how Pete Lestrel, of the University of California, Los Angeles, used one-dimensional Fourier transforms of the outline of a skull to compare many such outlines of many skulls. The method involves decomposing the complex curve (wave) forming the outline of the skull, through a one-dimensional Fourier transform, into the many simpler curves (waves) of which it is composed.

My use of the word 'wave' comes from the idea of music: decomposing complex sound waves into their simpler harmonics. This was a start, but it did not answer the direct question. I wanted to compare two-dimensional patterns or textures with one another. Yet two-dimensional waves seemed too difficult.

Someone, Somewhere, Has the Answer!

I discovered, of course, that this was already being done by many investigators in totally non-anatomical fields. For example, the first pictures from the moon needed to be cleaned up. Defence department aerial photographs (originally classified) needed to be analyzed. Structures of oil-bearing rocks (originally private) were important to the big oil companies. Even differences in the veins of leaves (of little interest to most of us) were important to botanists.

All of these problems had been tackled using various two-dimensional mathematical methods (called Walsh transforms, Hadamard-Walsh transforms and Hadamard transforms). I struggled for a year trying to understand them, to see if I could use them to characterize internal bone structure.

I thought these transforms were all different. Any 'real mathematician' would have laughed at me (they probably did!). But real mathematicians know, almost by 'osmosis', that they all belong in a single overarching mathematical set called the Karhunen Loeve series.

I went for two-dimensional Fourier transforms first. But I was immediately stymied because the mathematics of the two-dimensional Fourier transform, with its double integral, quite apart from being beyond me, was also beyond the computers of that time.

It was beyond me only, however, until the realization dawned upon me that two-dimensional Fourier analysis did not have to be done computationally; it could be done optically using a laser.

I realized then that what a lens does to a ray of light passing through it is to perform a Fourier transform on it. What, as a student, I understood as the focus of the light was also the Fourier transform of the information in the light stemming from the original picture. Add a second lens after the focus, and the light returns its image. This is the basis of any microscope. Any of my histological colleagues, especially those working with the then newly developed electron microscopes, would have known this almost intuitively. But microscopy had rather escaped me (which might seem peculiar to one educated as an anatomist).

But all this would have been useless to me without accidental collegial help, and this is, perhaps, almost the most important element of research!

Thus, one day, I was visiting a botanical statistical colleague, Peter Neeley, who had just moved from Chicago to Kansas (Kansas State Geological Survey). Peter said,

"Come and see what John Davis is doing."

"John Davis is an industrial geologist! Why should I see what he is doing?"

was my initial thought.

But my interest was piqued.

John Davis was looking at thin sections of rocks using an optical bench with a ruby laser, producing optical Fourier transforms. As soon as I saw John's rock sections and his transforms, I knew that my sections and radiographs of bone would be excellent subjects for such analysis.

John Davis was tickled pink and quickly produced the first colored transforms from my bones.

Of course, the optical bench he was using was (a) 22 feet long and (b) so susceptible to vibration that even a lorry going by outside would disturb it such that it had to be recalibrated all over again. When, later, I wanted one, my Dean offered me a room created by building a wall lengthwise along the center of a wide corridor: a space for a 22-foot-long optical bench!

At this point, another colleague, engineer Harold Pincus of the University of Milwaukee, came into the picture. He had folded the 22-foot bench into a small 3×3×3-foot box using mirrors. He was also giving a course in Milwaukee on its use. I took the course, bought one of these boxes, and I was away. Some colleagues laughed at my work, saying 'it was all done by mirrors'.

Inside an Ape's Spine: Rectangles and Honeycombs!

I first looked at sections (therefore two-dimensional pictures) of vertebrae, followed by lateral radiographs of vertebrae in a full study with MD/PhD Chicago student Harry Yang (later a Chicago surgeon). Radiographs are also two-dimensional — even if shadows — cast by x-rays, of three-dimensional objects. The pattern of shadows of bony spicules inside the vertebrae seemed to be a right-angled network in chimpanzees and gorillas, as well as in humans. There was nothing new here; we could see that by just looking at the chimpanzee radiograph of Figure 10.1.

However, when we examined a radiograph of the orang utan, which is not apparently much different from the chimpanzee, the transform implied a honeycomb structure (also Figure 10.1).

It was so different that I checked it by actually cutting sections of the bones (with permission). The orang utan section

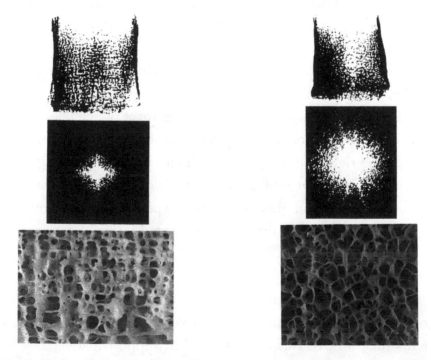

Figure 10.1: Above, radiographs of chimpanzee and orang utan vertebrae: though different, both seem to show approximately right-angled patterns. Middle, the left Fourier transform (chimpanzee) implies a right-angled pattern, but the right transform (orang utan) implies elements at many different angles. Below, cut sections: the chimpanzee (left) truly is a right-angled network; the orang utan (right) is actually more like a honeycomb.

showed exactly the honeycomb pattern predicted by the Fourier transform, but was largely hidden to visual inspection of the radiographs (Figure 10.1 yet again). How could the orang utan have such a different architecture?

Consideration of the peculiarities of behavior in orang utans suggests an answer. Unlike the other apes, orang utans have extremely varied postures and activities when in the trees. Orang utans have feet that are 'hands'. They can, thus, hang by one, two, three or all four 'hands' in all combinations, at all different angles, at all different times! In lectures, I had sometimes entertained the students by mimicking the four-limbed activity of the orang utan: raising one arm, then the other, then one foot, with the students expectantly waiting for me to raise my other foot!

Chimpanzees do not do this much. Humans (except circus acrobats!) not at all.

The maximum and minimum stresses are at right angles in any part of any one vertebrae at any one moment (by definition) and go with the right-angled spicules of bone. But, in the orang utan with a very wide range of activities, their orientations must vary much more over time than in the other species. The best overall supporting structure in the orang utan would, thus, be an architecture that is also varied in all directions — a honeycomb-like arrangement.

After all, if we wanted to support loads mainly in one direction, we would use a structure with vertical and horizontal elements (like a box). But if we wanted to support loads acting in many different directions over time, we might best choose a honeycomb (or bubble-wrap) structure. Certainly, in sending my grandmother's best china through the mail, with all the many ways in which postal workers drop it, I would use bubble wrap or some equivalent capable of bearing stresses in all directions!

Our ideas seemed acceptable. We had no difficulty publishing in top science journals (*Science*, USA; *Zoological Society*, London).

From Bone Structure in Apes to Human Osteoporosis!

It was, however, when we later came to apply this technology to examining spongy bone in human disease (osteoporosis) that we ran into problems. By then I was working with Alanah Buck, a PhD student at the University of Western Australia (who later became a forensic anthropologist with the West Australian Police).

At this time, too, we had moved from optical Fourier transforms to computer Fourier transforms.

This technology indicated very clearly (Figure 10.2) that the spongy bone networks in menopausal and older women were

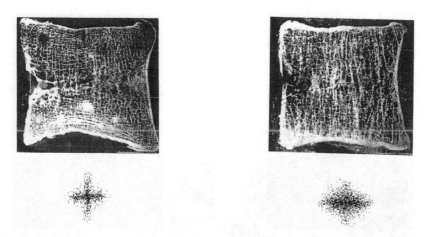

Figure 10.2: Top left, radiograph of section of vertebrae from a 45-year-old man, and top right, of a 45-year-old woman. Below are the corresponding Fast Fourier transforms.

The man shows a cruciate transform, a mainly right-angled pattern.
The woman shows a horizontally elongated pattern with longer vertical bony elements than horizontal (Fourier analyses are inverse functions). This is precisely what we see in her section, and she had a degree of osteoporosis.

different than in young women and most men. (Though by the time men were 80 years old, they too might have spongy bone networks like those in older women; it is only the timing that is different — fascinating information about an important disease process!)

Today's studies show us what osteoporotic bone actually looks like (Figure 10.3).

More importantly, however, we found that the new technique was sensitive enough to show an unusual arrangement in one specimen from a young woman of 25 years (Figure 10.4).

Of course, most young women do not have osteoporosis. But this individual had the initial stigmata of it in the right upper quadrant alone! This is where, in older women, osteoporotic fractures often first occur.

In other words, our technology could possibly detect the beginnings of osteoporosis. Of course, this young woman did not have osteoporosis; but she seemed to have its beginnings.

Today's studies show us what the bone actually looks like

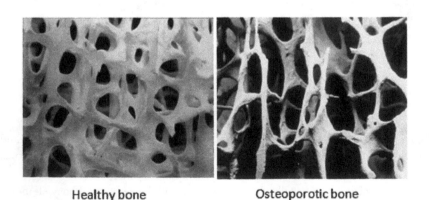

Healthy bone　　　　**Osteoporotic bone**

Figure 10.3: Actual normal and osteoporotic bone.

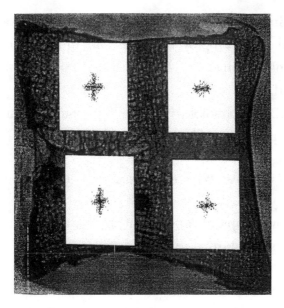

Figure 10.4: Fourier transforms for each quadrant of a section in a particular 25-year-old woman. Three of the transforms are cruciate as in young men. But the fourth quadrant, top right, shows a picture reminiscent of that in older menopausal osteoporotic women (compare with Figure 10.2).

This could be wonderful. By finding this in a particular individual, we could suggest lifestyle changes and advise drinking milk, taking up exercise, losing weight, quitting smoking, and, later, if indicated, hormone replacement therapy, and later still, new drugs that have come along. All might delay or even prevent osteoporosis!

Of course, this could not have applied here because these sections had been obtained post mortem, with permission, from known sexed and aged individuals from road accidents!

Why Was There a Problem?

Though we had no difficulty publishing the bone findings on apes in top science journals, we could never get the osteoporosis ideas on humans into medical journals. The work was always rejected because it did not employ the new and much more expensive DEXA technology involving bone density scans that had, by that time, evolved.

The DEXA technology was 'the gold standard' and our work was consistently rejected because it did not use it!

Do 'gold standards' stop new thoughts, new work and new ideas?

I am now happy to report that, today, thirty years later, the earlier studies are starting to be referenced.

More to the point, however, even newer computational methods are being used to investigate pattern, especially textures, in the three-dimensional images of spongy bone. Techniques such as tomograms, CAT scans, MRIs, and especially the functional versions of these, allow totally new information to be garnered.

Second: 'Accepted Wisdoms' and Fossils, Teeth and Sex!

While in California, I wrote a book titled *Fossils, Teeth and Sex*. I have a colleague who said he read the whole thing looking for the pieces about sex! But the story has an interesting beginning that is nothing to do with fossils and teeth.

In Los Angeles, I was working with Dr. Robin Crompton, then of the Chinese University of Hong Kong (but later Professor of Anatomy in Liverpool University, UK, and now Emeritus). I was also working with a research associate at the University of Southern California, Dr. Susan Lieberman (later, Director of Wild Life and Environment, Washington, DC). And I had a real artist, Erika Oller (who also worked with David Hockney); she was superb at sketching animals and anatomies.

Initially, we were working on relating my anatomical muscle and bone data in primates to Robin's fieldwork data on primate locomotion, environment and diet. Susan had a background in tropical ecology, the milieu within which these animals lived. In addition, she was accomplished at applying computer methods at which, by that time, I was becoming more and more rusty. She was, thus, an ideal third collaborator. Erika Oller pictured the animals beautifully, with the most living eyes, to illustrate our studies. The final result was a book that we all very much enjoyed writing: *Animal Lifestyles and Anatomies: The Case of the Prosimian Primates*. (Prosimians is what they were called then!)

However, the curious mixture of fossils, teeth and sex started from my attempts to obtain a salary for Susan and payment for Erika. This included getting an internal grant at the University of Southern California for a semester-long faculty seminar to develop an undergraduate course entitled, 'Similarities and Differences between the Sexes: Biological, Anthropological, Sociological and Psychological Approaches'. Susan and I were, of course, the biological individuals. I was able to recruit several other pairs of academics working in each of the other disciplines: anthropology, social science, and psychology. We got the grant!

Our first seminar was total disaster. Everyone came with prepared positions and everyone was talking in their own jargon. There was even a fight over the words 'sex' and 'gender'! It was actually a very angry meeting. I wondered if I had made a terrible mistake doing it at all.

However, over the next couple of meetings we all calmed down considerably. We all started to appreciate each other's points of view. We all started to discuss and collaborate instead of fight. In the end, the seminar was highly successful. But it seemed to us that the topic was not yet ready for an undergraduate course. The first course would have to be at the graduate level.

Sexual Dimorphism(?)

The entire idea of teaching about sexual differences arose because I had become involved in studies of biological sexual dimorphism (as biologists called it then) in monkeys and apes. First, sexual dimorphism was obviously not two separate conditions (small dimorphism, large dimorphism), but rather a spectrum running the gamut from small degrees in some species (e.g., humans) to very large degrees in others (e.g., orang utans and gorillas). Everyone knew this. (Today we know even more: the very term implying a dichotomy is incorrect.)

But in those days, for such studies, one needed large samples and quantitative data. The most extensive data one can get are measurements of teeth. Museums don't have many whole skeletons, but they do have many skulls and, hence, very many teeth. This was good; teeth are a body part that usually shows sexual dimorphism. Everyone knows the large canine differences between male and female gorillas compared to small differences between men and women.

What we found, of course, was that, even among teeth, there was no single dimorphism; there were several.

But the main problems came, as it seems they often do, when we tried to study fossils. We do not necessarily know the sex of a fossil tooth. Can we assess it, even if only approximately?

Teeth Have No Gonads!

Teeth are by far the commonest fossils. So, thanks to Professor Wu Ru Kang (Academia Sinica), I could examine measurements of more than two thousand fossil teeth from Lufeng and Guangxi. I was able to compare them with those of modern apes and humans (thanks to data from Bruce Gelvin, University of California, Northridge, Gene Albrecht, University of Southern California, and Clifford Wilcox, Orthodontist in Pasadena). I also examined data from the literature for further fossil and subfossil species.

Let us look at the Chinese fossils first. There were two ways to examine sexual dimorphism on the isolated Chinese fossil teeth. The first was to accept the diagnosis of sex as provided by our Chinese colleagues and examine their differences!

But how did our Chinese colleagues know? Who can 'sex' a tooth? They have no gonads!

Thus, when I first examined the overall distributions of tooth measurements (Figure 10.5), I found an approximately bell-shaped curve (which is what one might expect).

But when I examined the data by sex (based on my Chinese colleagues' determination of sex), I found that the distributions for each 'sex' were skewed in the opposite directions (Figure 10.6).

In other words, the smaller ones had been designated females, the larger, males.

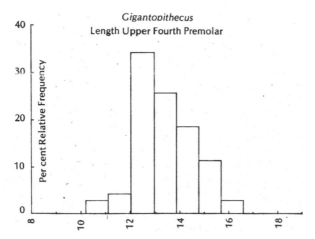

Figure 10.5: An example from Gigantopithecus. Given rather small numbers of specimens, the distribution, though a bit skewed, is approximately normal!

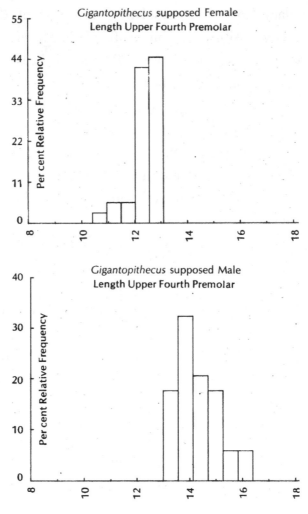

Figure 10.6:   Distributions of a particular measurement (length upper fourth premolar) for 'supposed' female and male teeth. Each supposed sex has the form of one half of a normal distribution; a totally unlikely situation!

This was confirmed when we examined the same data without presuming sex (Figure 10.7). It is clear that the 'supposed sexes' of Figure 10.6 are just one half, each, of the overall distribution of Figure 10.7! (Incidentally, plots like this do not mean there is no bimodality; it just means they do not show it.)

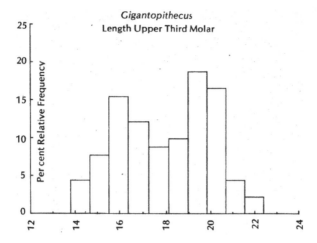

Figure 10.7: Distributions of lengths of upper third molar in all specimens of *Gigantopithecus*. The distribution is bimodal with a big difference between the modes. Is this marked sexual dimorphism?

In contrast, however, it was possible to find some teeth with quite different distributions. Figure 10.7 shows the distribution for the length of the upper third molar tooth *(this analysis was done without trying to guess the 'sex' of the teeth)*.

Immediately, the findings for *Gigantopithecus* became extra interesting. They not only imply very large dimorphism, but also roughly *equal numbers of each sex!* This is quite different from the large dimorphic apes (many more females than males). But we had only a few specimens, so this may be accidental.

The many teeth from Lufeng were a very different matter. They had first been sorted as two separate genera by our Chinese hosts and given, at that time, the names *Ramapithecus* and *Sivapithecus*. (Later the names changed because a single name, *Lufengpithecus*, became applied to them). That is, they became a single species with sexual dimorphism.

I therefore examined the distributions of tooth dimensions (Figure 10.8) for these *apparently* clearly separate sexes. However,

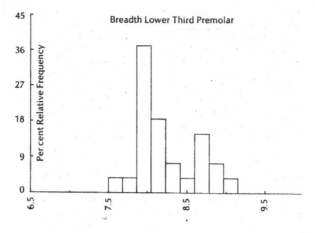

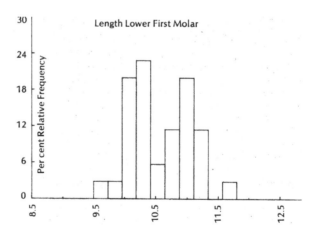

Figure 10.8:   Upper frame: tooth lengths of the lower third premolar in what were judged as the males of *Lufengpithecus* (the 'old' *Sivapithecus* specimens) are **unequally** bimodal. Lower frame: tooth lengths of the lower first molar in what were judged as the females of *Lufengpithecus* (the old *Ramapithecus* specimens) are **equally** bimodal.

instead of finding an approximately normal distribution for each 'sex', as one would expect, I found that each 'sex' was, itself, bimodal!

Not only that, but the numbers of specimens in each mode varied! In the bigger group, there were more small specimens and fewer large ones. In the smaller group, there were equal numbers of small and large specimens.

I was therefore forced to assume that these could not be the two sexes of one species. They must be something else. *We clearly do not have a single species.*

But Figure 10.8 does not show the only possibility. There are a number of others. For example, the two sets of double-peaked distributions might each belong across the groups instead of within the groups; that is, large dimorphism in each of two species, or three species one with dimorphism and one without, and so on!

The 'accepted wisdom' ignored these findings.

One reason is that some workers did not understand what had been done. They seemed to think I had identified the sexes before analysis (which is impossible). They thought this, even though my methods made it clear that I examined the data without defining sex.

A second reason stemmed from the fact that shortly after our studies, the general company of anthropologists had renamed the entire collection as the single group of *Lufengpithecus*. Again, therefore, the 'conventional wisdom' came into play. Most investigators '*knew*' there was only one group (*Lufengpithecus*) and that, therefore, there could be *only two sexes!*

This is not the first time that sex and species differences have been confused!

My suggestion was, therefore, not just incorrect, but damned! Could we check this out in any way?

Application to Known Ape and Human Teeth

I decided to test these findings by using present-day apes and humans where I knew (from field, museum and dental records) which tooth comes from which sex, and in which species. I could then compare results from these known species and known sex specimens, with the results obtained if I 'pretended' I did not know species and sex for these data.

Moreover, I could also do such tests on samples from the living species where I deliberately chose equal numbers of each sex or where I deliberately chose fewer males than females (to see if I could identify these two different situations).

The results were unequivocal. I could easily identify large versus small sexual dimorphism. Furthermore, and this is critical, I could also easily identify situations: where I had chosen the numbers of each sex to be equal, and where I had deliberately made the numbers of each sex unequal.

In all these cases, I was 'sex-blinded' (like being 'double-blinded'!), pretending that I did not know the sexes of the specimens from the living species.

But let's be clear what else was in this study. Could these data be biased? These species were largely from museum collections of today's species, and such samples can be biased for many reasons. For example, in the old days, collectors frequently 'collected' more males than females (because they were larger and more greatly prized), or they might collect more female skulls because female skulls were easier to get. These are the kinds of biases collectors might have to struggle with.

But fossil collections, though they may be biased by many factors, are not biased by collectors' habits. Quite the reverse, the fossil hunter takes every fossil that can be found! Biased the sex subsamples in fossils are likely to be, but not by 'human' selection!

The 'sex-blind' analyses of the teeth of extant species allowed understanding of the situations in extinct species. Thus, subfossil orang utans (very much like today's orang utans) were similar to fossil australopithecines in having double peaks for many of the teeth, and with more specimens in the smaller peak (more females than males?). In contrast, subfossil gibbons (like today's humans and gibbons) were similar to fossil humans. And in those few specific teeth that had double peaks, there were equal numbers in each peak (equal numbers of females and males?).

The similarity of the subfossil orang utans and subfossil gibbons to their present-day analogues, modern orang utans and modern gibbons, implies that the subfossil assessments for fossils like australopithecines, with no living analogues, may also be correct.

Once again, these data, their statistics, and the ideas that stem from them have been ignored. *They contravene the accepted wisdom.* But these findings are suspiciously suggestive!

Third: 'Best Practices' and the Biomechanics of Bones

Understanding the anatomical structure of bones relates to understanding the mechanical functions of bones. Thus, a very old theory was the 'trajectorial theory of bone architecture', based initially upon the well-known 18th century comparison of engineering and biological structures. It showed that the right-angled network of stresses that can be calculated as due to load bearing in an engineering object (a crane) is similar to the right-angled network of bony architecture that can be seen in a biological object (the

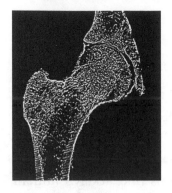
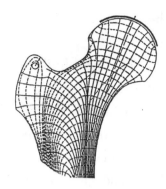

Figure 10.9: Left, the pattern of bony spicules in a section of the femur; right, the pattern of stresses calculated as existing in a loaded femur. The similarity is obvious!

femur). The theory was that, in some way, the mechanical stresses might be responsible for the bony architectures (Figure 10.9).

Further, studying mechanical strains is also very old. Brewster, in the early 1800s, had realized that if certain transparent materials were stressed and then examined under polarized light, colored bands could be seen. The colors, like a rainbow, showed the strain.

The only transparent material available to Brewster was glass. His models were fragile — under load, they might show half a band and then break. He persevered and founded experimental strain analysis.

Nowadays there are many such materials, such as perspex and macrolon. Some of these are so sensitive that they show many colored bands even under very low loads. They confirm the relationship between right-angled architectures and right-angled strains.

However, it was only as I started to think about the implications of three dimensions that I had doubts. Not about the general idea that architectures and mechanics are causally associated, but doubts about the direct application of two-dimensional pictures to three-dimensional cases.

Stresses and Strains in Bone

The two-dimensional case says that, at any particular point in a bone (or any other structure), the local stress distorts (strains) a tiny circle of bone into a tiny ellipse. The long and short diameters of the ellipse, at right angles to one another, indicate where the equal diameters of the original circle have been maximally compressed (in one direction) and elongated (tensed, in the other direction at right angles to the first; Figure 10.10).

Throughout the two-dimensional section of the whole bone, we can envision the strains as a network of maximum compressions and elongations aligned at right angles throughout the section. This is the basis of the trajectorial theory of bone architecture described above.

However, let us look at some examples in going from two dimensions to three (Figure 10.11).

Once again, a departure into art helps us further understand what is happening.

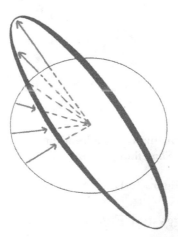

Figure 10.10: A small unloaded circle of bone at any point in the bone deformed into an ellipse by loading. Some of the diameters of the original circle are elongated, others compressed.

**A simple minded change to
three dimensions suggests the following:**

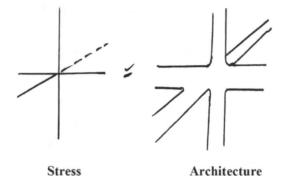

Stress   **Architecture**

**This is what happens in a building!
But is it what happens in bone?**

Figure 10.11:   Stress in architecture.

Thanks to Art (Escher) we might think bone is like this:

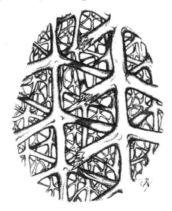

**Though this picture is like a building, it is not like a bone
Something else is happening?**

Figure 10.12:   An Escher picture!

Escher has suggested Figure 10.12 as a possible structure. Indeed, this is what is seen in a building, but it is not the way it is in a bone!

Sections of the body of a vertebra can show the differences in Figure 10.13.

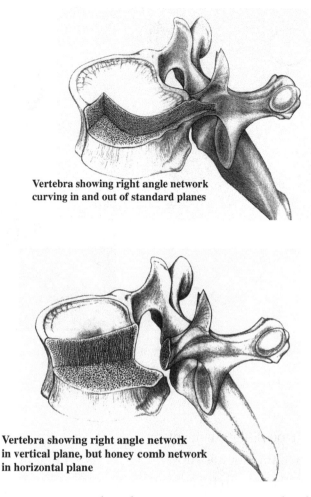

**Vertebra showing right angle network
curving in and out of standard planes**

**Vertebra showing right angle network
in vertical plane, but honey comb network
in horizontal plane**

Figure 10.13: Two vertebrae showing patterns in various angles of section.

Further, if we look at stresses at a point in dimensions at right angles to one another (the traditional sections of histology), it is not logically possible for all three sections to show ellipses with one compressed and one tensed diameter. One possibility is for all the original circles to be compressed in all directions; that is, all with compressed diameters. One might find this in an abyssal fish under compression of tons of water, or, over time, in a spherical bone such as the head of the thigh bone (Figure 10.14).

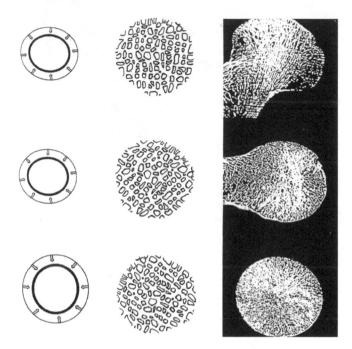

Figure 10.14:   Stresses (and strains) in each of the three dimensions in the head of the femur (first column), theoretical architectural elements to fit with this (second column) and the actual architectural elements (third column).

Another possibility is in places in the skeleton with regions where mechanical analysis shows zero stresses in all directions. In these places, there is no bone.

This is most obvious in a cow tibia, where there is not only no bone but actually a fluid-containing cyst marked with an arrow (Figure 10.15).

It is also evident in many other bones where there are areas of no trabeculae (e.g., special regions in the heel bone and in the neck of the femur, long recognized by radiologists).

There are even the possibilities when there are two ellipses with compression and tension at right angles to one another (Figure 10.16).

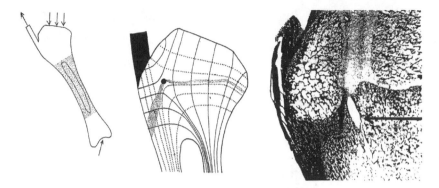

Figure 10.15: Left, model of a cow's tibia showing a black dot in the region of no stress; right, section of a cow's tibia showing region (arrowed) of a fluid-filled cyst at that position.

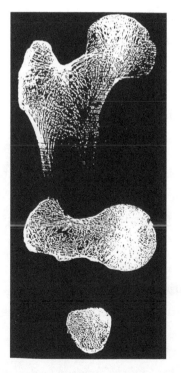 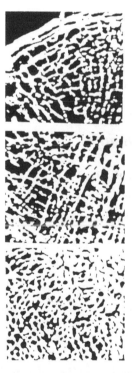

Figure 10.16: Actual bony spicules in three sections of the head and neck of the femur. Two of the planes have the spicules organized as a right-angled network; the third plane has spicules in all directions.

The opposite of Figure 10.16 is an example where one section of a bone shows the right-angled compression/tension network while each of the other two shows tension alone. This may be seen in a bony structure that is a thin plate, with the thinness of the plate being in the double-tension direction. One such example is the thin plate of the shoulder blade, and it is indeed the case that in some situations, the shoulder blade is so thin that it may have a foramen (a hole) in it covered by membrane (a tension-bearing material). Other examples are in the skull of some reptiles and the obturator part of the human pelvis where, again, there is a hole (foramen), but one that is covered by a tension-bearing collagenous sheet. Where there is only tension, there is only fascia!

The conclusion to all this is that it is not a simple matter to go from two dimensions to three; yet three dimensions are the 'real world' case!

Further 'Best Practices': Measuring Bones using Landmarks

Another problem involving the extra complexity of three dimensions came about as the morphometrics in which I was involved in the middle of last century (the 'old morphometrics') was mutated (by others) into the 'new morphometrics' at the end of the last century and into this.

Questions raised by consideration of biological form and pattern are actually very old. In the time of the Ancients, Pythagoras wrote:

> "All things have form, all things are form, and all forms can be defined by numbers."

Another 2,000 years were to pass until the appearance of D'Arcy Thompson's seminal book, *On Growth and Form* (1917). In this he wrote,

> *"We begin by describing the shape of an object in the simple words of common speech.*
>
> *We end by defining it in the precise language of mathematics."*

Fifteen years after Thompson, Julian Huxley recognized his debt to Thompson's work, and in *Problems of Relative Growth* he wrote:

> *"Among many morphologists . . . there appears to still linger distrust . . . of quantitative expression . . . yet without quantitative expression, we should largely be theorizing in the air."*

Bones can be studied by measuring from landmarks. What is a landmark? We can all recognize by eye such landmarks as the point of the chin or the prominence of the cheek. Such were the basis of earlier attempts to measure form. The more landmarks that could be identified on a bone, the more information could be obtained about that bone's shape.

This led eventually to the absurdity of a study that involved more than 4,000 anatomical landmarks on a single skull! Presumably the investigator was so worn out by this activity that it was never repeated on any other skull. What, therefore, did it achieve?

Measurements first 'measured' biological form by being the distance between pairs of landmarks (i.e., *size*). Later followed ratios of two sizes (i.e., *proportions*). Later still, the computer allowed combinations of measurements from many landmarks, characterizing *shape*.

In pre-Darwinian biology, the information from corresponding landmarks within an organism was thought to give description: the structural *Bauplan* of ideal types, description but not evolution. With the onset of ideas of evolution, the correspondence of landmarks was thought to show differences between the various descendants (from ancestors). Modern evolutionary biology provides three additional ideas. The correspondences of landmarks may relate to:

parts that, themselves, become changed during development and growth of the same individual (therefore during 'physiological time'), parts *that compared with other parts* in different species *have changed* over evolutionary time (therefore during 'deep time', as it has been called); and to the fact that these *two changes are present together*. In these cases, information content derives from adding change to structure.

Modern functional anatomy adds yet other ideas. Further correspondences of landmarks derive from recognizing the effects of animal functions. This may result from correspondences:

between parts changed in position in the same individual (e.g., *due to movement*, kinetics);

between parts changed in form in between individuals (e.g., *due to function*, mechanics);

between parts with *different developmental origins*, but with *similar functions*;

between parts with the *same developmental origins*, but subserving *different functions*; and

between parts involved in any two or more of these.

So, it's complex.

Measuring Without Landmarks! A Totally New 'Best Practice'

How can we characterize anatomical regions where there are very few anatomical landmarks of any kind? That is: how can we describe skullcaps, eggs, or fruits (largely featureless)?

This has resulted in the idea of new forms of landmark ('semi-landmarks' where invented landmarks are interpolated between real ones, and 'sliding landmarks' where semi-landmarks are 'slid') to measure the shape of an object. Both are inventive and extremely useful.

Obviously, studies of measurements from developmental and growth landmarks might give information speaking to development or growth of the animal; studies of biomechanical landmarks might perhaps speak to function; studies of evolutionary landmarks perhaps to evolution. That all sounds simple. But of course, most landmarks play roles in more than a single category.

Professor Paul O'Higgins (UWA, UCL and York in sequence) and I had a series of discussions about this mixing of landmark types. We wondered what the implications might be for interpretation. We had such fierce arguments that I was afraid we would have a 'domestic'. Paul and I were close colleagues, have been close colleagues, had a close 'academic father' [Professor Eric Ashton] and, indeed, for most of our academic lives, have been associated across several institutions.

Our 'domestic' was eventually muted by appeal to another colleague: Fred Bookstein. As a result, Paul and I were able to publish together a paper that must have in it the most curious set of pictures of relationships between biological objects that I have ever seen. It examined the relationships of some skull landmarks from infants, adolescents and adults of, sequentially, chimpanzees, gorillas, and humans. It demonstrated that attention must be paid to these different landmark categories, and that they greatly affect interpretations (see another chapter). Of course, this was not a full and detailed study; it was merely a preliminary examination of the problems.

Better Standards, Unconventional Wisdoms and New Practices!

These three cases, osteoporotic disease, sexual dimorphism and bone shape, point to a number of problems in doing science. They show the importance of divorcing one's self from gold standards to allow for better standards, from accepted wisdoms to allow for unconventional wisdoms, and from best practices to allow for new practices.

The original ideas are not necessarily wrong. It is just that they *may* be wrong. But just being wrong is the least of it. It is being attached too closely to the original ideas that prevents us from seeing when they may be wrong, and we don't know it! That prevents us, in turn, from seeing better standards, unconventional wisdoms, and totally new practices.

Recognizing such 'straitjackets' is essential before we can possibly escape from them!

11 Chapter '0-Metrics': Finding What is Hidden!

The earlier studies showed that understanding bone forms and patterns visually (eye-balling) could be greatly improved through the use of measurement (and analysis). They gave better comparisons of form and sometimes revealed unexpected (hidden) suggestions about function. Of course, I loved to play the maverick. Although most of the studies were of today's bones where you can assess function in other ways, the results also suggested ideas about the function of yesterday's bones (fossils). We were calling our methods *'morphometrics'* as a shorthand descriptor.

Morphometrics was regarded as unorthodox in those early days. One student who used some of my statistical plots was ordered by her supervisor to *'de-Oxnardize'* her thesis. Since then, however, morphometrics has been increasingly vindicated. I am, thus, now beginning to look rather orthodox, possibly even out of touch! If so, however, it is not because I have conformed to others' orthodoxies, but rather that others found themselves conforming, through their own finds, their own researches, to my original *'unorthodoxies'*!

One of my delights in academia has been in reducing the seemingly insurmountable complexity of nature to simpler (often esthetically pleasing) patterns. Yet at the same time, by pushing the studies one more step, I have sometimes found that apparent simplicities may yield new and surprising complexities.

However, I did not develop these methods myself. I borrowed from toolkits already on the workbenches of others. These were the tools of data ordering, graphical display, biomechanical analysis and bioengineering as described in other chapters. As a young man, Fred Bookstein had reviewed my 1973 book (*Form and Pattern in Human Evolution*) and he commented:

"If Oxnard had not noted an approach here, either it was not worth noting, or it had been invented after 1973."

And he further said:

"Multivariate morphometrics, medial axis transforms, clustering techniques, Cartesian transformation grids, optical Fourier analysis and optical stress analysis — all were recapitulated in that short book as a potential toolkit for the study of form and pattern."

At first, my almost painful early attempts to find out what was hidden in individual measurements were visualized by making physical models.

My somewhat more painful attempts to understand hidden aspects of overall shape used D'Arcy Thompson's deformation of Cartesian coordinates, and they have since been improved beyond all recognition by many workers. These include Fred Bookstein and his biorthogonal grids, Pete Lestrel and his Fourier curves, Gene Albrecht and his thin plate splines, and perhaps, closest to me, Paul O'Higgins and his original toolkit: Morphologika.

These (and many other similar developments) revealed new *differences* between biological structures as a result of evolution. However, they could also show *changes* in structures as a result of growth, *deformations* of structures as altered by mechanical loads, and *positions* of structures as they changed during movement.

They could do all this not only within the variations of many specimens within a single universe of specimens, but also among the many different universes of specimens that might represent age cohorts, geographic communities, ecological guilds, species groups, evolutionary clades, and so on.

My especially painful early studies are now almost totally superseded by these new developments of many workers. Happily, however, I have been able to continue to participate through collaborations with students, ex-students and colleagues.

Form in the Skeleton: 'Osteo-metrics'

When I first applied multivariate technologies to bones, they seemed not only to demonstrate differences in form (which is what they were measuring), but also hinted at other types of difference. For example, the earliest studies of forelimb *form* seemed to separate species by estimates of forelimb *function* (see earlier, and Figures 11.1 and 11.2).

Studies of hindlimb form (Figure 11.3) gave a different but still functional result.

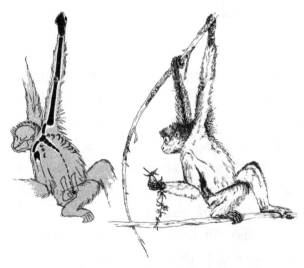

Figure 11.1: Cartoon showing the forelimb components that were measured.

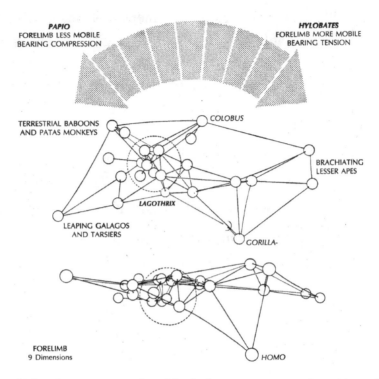

Figure 11.2:   Osteometric results of forelimb measurement analysis. Upper frame: theory of forelimb functions in nonhuman primates. Middle frame: osteometric result of forelimb measurements is a band that mirrors the theoretical band of forelimb use. Lower frame: the third dimension shows that the position of humans is unique.

In contrast to the spectrum of function in the upper limb (a band), the model of hindlimb function is a star (Figure 11.4, upper frame). The center of the star contains those many primates that utilize hindlimbs in regular quadrupedal modes. The various arms of the star are the species that utilize the lower limbs in more unusual modes (e.g., slow climbing: *loris*, leaping: *tarsius*, a different kind of leaping: *propithecus*, etc).

Parallel with the functional model is the osteometric result. Viewed from one angle, the nonhuman primates are indeed arranged in a star-shaped spectrum (Figure 11.4, middle frame).

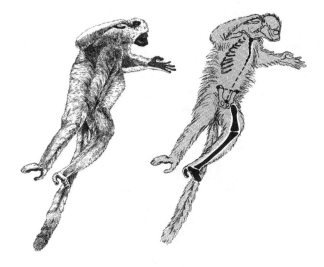

Figure 11.3: Cartoon showing the hindlimb components that were measured.

But another view of the morphometric result separates out humans (Figure 11.4, lowest frame).

Given the totally different functional results from fore-limbs and hind-limbs separately, I wondered what would be the result of adding limbs together: *aggregation.*

This result was quite different from that for either limb alone, as might be expected (Figures 11.5 and 11.6). It still seems heavily functional but in a different way, and appears to relate to degree of participation of each limb within locomotion. Forelimb-dominated species were placed together, hindlimb-dominated species likewise, and those species with approximately equal uses of both limbs, whatever the specific locomotor patterns of the different species, were placed together. All this was achieved without showing similarities relating to evolution. Even humans, as lower limb-dominated bipeds but presumably derived from forelimb-dominant antecedents, fitted at an appropriately unique place, converting the curved figure into the shape of a signet ring!

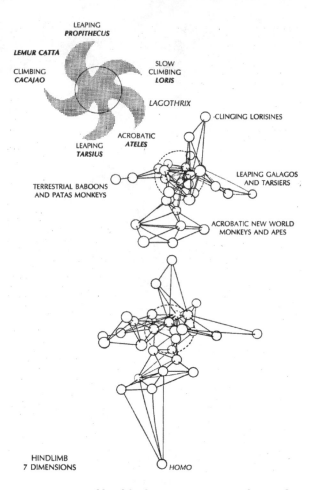

Figure 11.4:   Osteometrics of hind-limb measures. Upper frame: theory of usage of hind-limb in nonhuman primates is a star. Middle frame: osteometric result of separations of hind-limb measurements mirrors the theoretical model. Lower frame: a third view shows the position of humans is different from all the rest.

In complete contrast, however, was the effect of a *further level of aggregation*: adding measures of both limbs, abdomen and thorax, and neck and head (Figure 11.7). The parts that seemed to speak about function when examined locally now seemed to show evolution when examined globally.

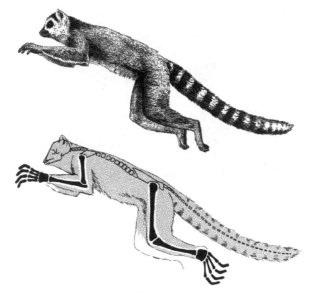

Figure 11.5: Cartoon of both limb components measured.

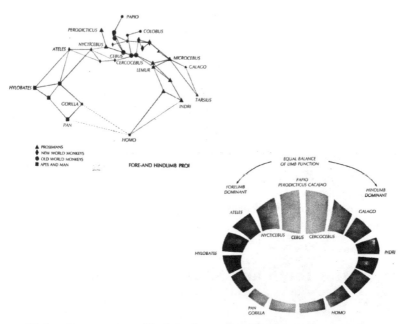

Figure 11.6: Osteometrics of both limbs combined and including humans seems to give a signet ring-shaped spectrum. Yet again, however, the spectrum seems to reflect function in primates. Maybe the summation of a band and a star give rise, mathematically, to a signet ring!

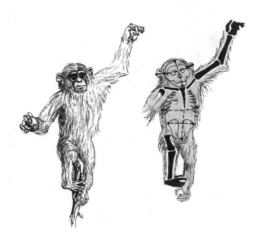

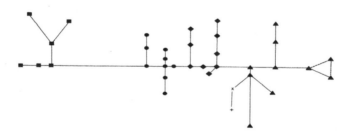

Figure 11.7:   All parts of the body combined (figured in the upper frame) give an osteometric result (minimum spanning tree: lower frame) that shows the species arranged as *per* their evolutionary relationships: squares = humans and apes, circles = old world monkeys, diamonds = new world monkeys, and triangles = prosimians (as they were called at the time).

Form in the Teeth and Skull: 'Odontometrics, Craniometrics'

We then went on to examine more complex areas like the teeth, jaws, face and cranium. In the jaws alone, there seemed to be only two levels of analysis in our investigations: individual tooth regions (i.e., molars, premolars, canines and incisors) and the dental battery as a whole.

At the *first level of analysis*, the individual tooth regions (not at all surprisingly) gave results that mirrored functions like chewing (*powerful dental batteries for the mastication of fibrous foods as compared with softer fruits*) and small or large sexual dimorphisms (*in accordance with facial comparisons of males and females*).

In contrast, however, at the *second level of analysis*, or the dental battery as a whole, the results mirrored ancient evolutionary relationships (e.g., placing humans with African chimpanzees and gorillas, and these three contrasting with Asian gibbons and orang utans).

But in the final examination of the more complex overall skull, we found three anatomical levels of analysis. *First*, most species separations seemed to be about simple size (a not-at-all surprising result). *Second*, there was separation of species-size differences from sex-size differences, indicating sexual dimorphism. Finally, *third*, we found that these first two sets of difference covered only about a third of the information content of the data. The additional two-thirds seemed to relate to developmental and evolutionary ideas about skull form.

Apart from helping to better understand living species, results like these have a special importance for studies of fossils which are mostly incomplete. This can scarcely be overemphasized. It suggests that attempts to understand results stemming from incomplete fossils, and therefore with only partial data, absolutely require an understanding of the effects of aggregation of data obtainable only from studies of complete forms (generally living).

This allows us to know **not only what data are missing**, but also **what interpretations are thereby excluded!**

Form in Soft Tissues: More 'O-metrics'

Many of the studies described above are relatively clear because they examine data from bones and teeth. Bones and teeth are hard tissues and can be measured to 0.2 of a millimeter. The resulting data are 'hard'. However, such analyses can also be applied to data from soft tissues. Measures from soft tissues are often much 'softer'.

Soft Tissues: Muscles

One example of a soft tissue is muscle — closely related functionally to the bones that they move. The closeness of that relationship allows data from muscles to be tested using data from bones.

For example, morphometric studies of shoulder, arm and hip muscles carried out in the 1980s provided information about function similar to that provided by morphometric studies of shoulder, arm and hip bones in the 1970s. These results enhanced the idea that the form of these bones reflected the functions of the muscles that move them.

But such muscle studies are inherently more difficult than bone studies, even if only because it is more difficult to get measurements about muscles in large numbers of specimens and species. As a result, I am not aware of any other major morphometric study of whole muscle data. In any case, the information from muscles is so clearly reflected in information from bones that these latter may be all that are required.

Thank goodness it never occurred to me to call these studies **my-o-metrics**. You can certainly carry an idea too far!

Even Softer Tissues: Brains

Of course, other soft materials can also be studied in this way. Thus, our studies then came to involve brains.

The earliest investigations of the sizes of brain parts showed, primarily, relationships with overall brain size and, indeed, overall body size as well. These studies (Stephan, Jerison, among many other investigators) were mainly carried out by examining variables one at a time (linear measures) and in pairs (ratios). They showed an almost complete relationship with size. They led, therefore, to concepts of increasing degrees of encephalization (in mammals) and increasing degrees of hominization (among primates). They were even sometimes (in humans) related by some workers to increasing degrees of 'intelligence'!

We confirmed the size relationship using morphometrics (as had many other investigators). Using Stephan's raw data (over 1,000 specimens of 40 or so mammalian species), we showed that the relative sizes of the brain parts of mammals, spanning several orders of magnitude (from the tiniest of insectivores and bats to humans), arranged the species along a primary axis that contains 98.4% of the morphometric information. This axis is correlated 96% with the size of the whole brain, and very nearly to a similar degree with the size of the entire body. Of course, everyone knew this!

However, more complex morphometric methods looking at variations within species as well as between species, and attempting to assess input-output relationships between brain parts, revealed a new story and gave several additional axes of separation.

In this, the work of Willem de Winter was critical and we called this **'neurometrics'**.

The supremacy of size in the first axis of the analysis of raw measurements of the brain is almost total.

But in these new multivariate analyses, more than a single axis was necessary to show the results. Several new axes were found and they showed very clear separations of groups of species with convergent lifestyles *irrespective of size*. Indeed, these lifestyle clusters, previously hidden, are far more interesting than the overall relationship with size!

Among bats for example, we found groups of species with similar lifestyles. Thus, all surface-gleaning bats fell together, all fish-eating bats fell together and all nectar-feeding bats fell together. And these three groups were irrespective of the fact that each contains species from both New and Old Worlds (separate for 30 or more millions of years).

We made similar findings for insectivores. All semi-aquatic species were neighbors, as were all burrowing species and all terrestrial species, separately, and this was again irrespective of their different degrees of evolutionary relationship.

These lifestyle associations were particularly clear in primates. Thus, among nonhuman primates, all species sharing forelimb-dominant modes of locomotion (and, of course, other lifestyle features that go with them) were tightly located within a space bounded by only three standard deviation units despite being comprised of species as different as great apes, lesser apes and prehensile tailed monkeys. These species were clearly and completely separated from all extensively hindlimb-dominant (leaping) primates. These latter lay in another tight locality of about four standard deviation units of extent. Further still, all those primate species with approximately equally combined fore- and hindlimb-dominated locomotion (quadrupedal running and climbing) lay intermediately between the aforementioned groups. (These species groups have been given here anatomical and locomotor titles for convenience, though, of course, many other lifestyle factors are part of such designations.)

However, there were more differences when we looked at humans! Three more higher axes separated humans from all other primates. When these axes were added (in a Pythagorean manner), humans differed from other primates by a staggering 22 standard deviation units.

This difference between humans and all other primates is expressed here as a 'quantitative distance'. However, because it is a multidimensional distance dependent upon all 19 brain variables, it is actually more of a measure of 'qualitative difference' in the organization of brains.

We showed that it is due to independent increases in humans of the neocortex, cerebellum, striatum and diencephalon as compared with the medulla combined with independent reductions of the midbrain, schizocortex and diencephalon as compared with the neocortex. These are relationships between and within the middle and upper brain parts.

Do these organizational differences relate to human expansions of the highest levels of the hierarchy of voluntary activities, as well as increased capacities to plan and control complex strategies (see another chapter)?

Very Soft Data, Greater Complexity, Behavior: Niche-metrics

As our investigations expanded, so we named further new 'o-metrics'. One of these arose when we tried to understand relationships between anatomical structure and field behavior (work with Robin Crompton and Sue Sima Lieberman, see earlier).

We called these studies **'niche-metrics'**, not knowing that this term was already being used in a different way in behavioral biology. Never mind; our term fits our study extremely well — they provided us with direct comparisons between measurement of anatomies in the laboratory (bones) and how the animals lived in the field (niche).

In these investigations, we found that analyses of data about locomotor activities, arboreal environments and dietary choices provided arrangements of the animals (prosimian primates) that made sense in terms of the niches that the animals inhabit and, therefore, also the lifestyles that they display. We also showed, however, that these niche-metric results were parallel to prior osteometric studies of their anatomies.

And we did not find this just once, but five times within each of the five sets of animals that we studied, thus constituting a very robust finding. It opens new vistas for studying living species and makes possible new reverse predictions from fossil anatomies to fossil lifestyles!

These parallels are entirely at the functional level. This is just like other first-level investigations described in this chapter.

However, another way of examining these same data provides arrangements of the animals in relation to the families into which they are usually classed. The Malagache primate known as the aye-aye was a much greater outlier in this study than it should be if it were just another lemur. This result even gave rise to a publication, 'The Uniqueness of Daubentonia' (Daubentonia: aye-aye, Figure 11.8).

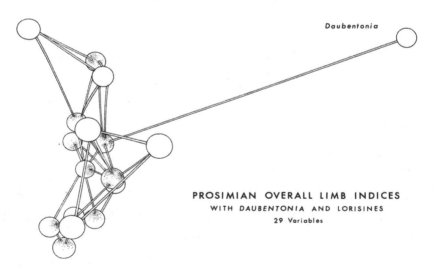

Daubentonia

PROSIMIAN OVERALL LIMB INDICES
WITH *DAUBENTONIA* AND LORISINES
29 Variables

Figure 11.8:   Daubentonia is separated from all other lorisines in a different dimension from those separating the other lorisines. This is a separation reminiscent of the separation of humans from all other primates (see above).

In other words, in addition to the functional relationships just described, these analyses showed relationships that seemed to relate to evolution. These latter analyses broke niche linkages between convergent forms and revealed linkages between evolutionarily related groups!

Yet Even 'Softer' Data: Form of Ships, or 'Ship-O-metrics'

Because Willem de Winter's partner was working on the reconstruction of old Dutch ships (in the Maritime Museum in Fremantle), we came to apply measurements and analyses to ships! Of course, we could not measure the old ships — very few were available.

But paintings and sketches, made not only by professional artists but also by sailors needing something to do while in port, could be 'measured'. Such sketches were obviously only approximate and contained no absolute measurements, but they give **relative** proportions obtained from ships in different artistic perspectives! We were familiar with such **relative** data because most of our biological measurements had come from colleagues who had only been able to provide **relative** proportions. So, we already had some knowledge there.

Hence (tongue in cheek), we called these studies '**shipo-metrics**'. But our results were useful; they classified the vessels in ways that seemed to correlate with their nautical uses!

Believe It or Not: 'Nose-O-metrics'

I've even seen a paper on nasal form ('**nose-o-metrics**'?) for researching the wild southern male elephant seal using image analysis and geometric morphometrics!

The Softest Data of All: 'Make-Believe-O-metrics'!

Some of these ideas could be tested in what, for me, was a relatively new mode of investigation. Could we model what goes on in evolution? Such modelling does not tell us what happened, but it might give insights into the kinds of things that might have happened! And possibly also, and this is even more important, into what was extremely unlikely to have happened. Is it possible to gain some insight into the effects of the many 'accidental' factors that may intrude into evolutionary assessments?

For example, most of the species that have ever existed are never found. Can we assess the effect of not taking them into account in estimating lineages from the few fossils we know?

For example, again, though we know that interbreeding and migration must have occurred many times in evolution, can we estimate their effects on lineages?

For example, once more, though we have information from mitochondrial DNA (females) and Y chromosome studies (males), do we understand the differences between lineages observed through matrilines and patrilines, and within and between species?

For example, finally, many 'characters' used in studying fossils are evaluated as simply binary: 'primitive' or 'derived' characters. Do we understand the effects of treating them this way when, in actuality, they are continuous and complex, and with many underlying causations?

A start has been made in examining questions like these using mathematical mimicry of evolutionary events (Figure 11.9). This, indeed, is **'Make-Believe-O-metrics'**.

Although such studies cannot tell us what did happen, they can tell us what might have happened, and they can certainly indicate what is unlikely to have happened, even sometimes, what

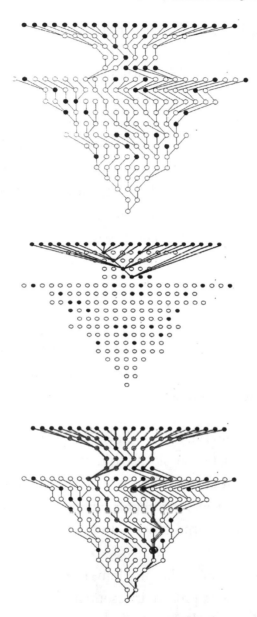

Figure 11.9: Upper frame: An evolutionary model showing relationships between fossil species (solid dots) and species never found as fossils with a bottleneck near the present day.

Middle frame: Result based upon cladistic analysis of data for each fossil — the bottleneck seems to produce a common ancestor close to the present day.

Lower frame: The actual relationships in the model. There are actually three lineages, and the overall common ancestor (large black ring) is far back in time!

could not have happened! (The principal worker here was physicist Ken Wessen as detailed in another chapter.)

Such studies imply, for instance, that whenever we study the 'characters' of fossil and living forms, we are likely to be two, three, or even many times too recent in our assessments of common ancestry. But when we allow for factors such as, in this model, speciation, extinction and interbreeding, we obtain very different relationships, with many fossils being nothing to do with lineages leading to the present day, with some other fossils indicating much older assessments of common ancestry.

It is obvious that assessments of fossils can never be absolutely correct. That follows inevitably from the partial nature of any investigation where we do not have access to all species, or all characters, and so on. That is not, however, the problem. The problem is that we need to have estimates of how right or wrong such judgments may be. Studies like these are now suggesting that conventional estimates may be far more wrong than we think.

O-metrics as defined here thus have the potential to aid in the understanding of data complexity to degrees greater now than at any time in the last century. The new forms of data and the new technologies are particularly important, as are the ways in which they uncover new interpretations. But so, too, are a number of other factors.

A clear definition of the problem, rather than a 'let's look at some data, any data' approach, is essential.

Careful thought about the design of observations and the levels of analysis are both especially useful. Such studies can go beyond hard tissues (e.g., bones and teeth — most easily obtained) into soft tissues (e.g., muscle), soft organs (e.g., the brain) and into 'even softer' data (e.g., those of behavior, diet, environment), and even into the totally invented data of 'make-believe-O-metrics' (just how soft are they?). Such studies are certainly fun and may be useful.

What other **'O-metrics'** might there be?

Chapter 12 International Links: Especially China!

Professor (then Dr.) Peter Lisowski, an experienced career anatomist in Birmingham, had special expertise in mentoring overseas and mature medical students. The time came when he temporarily helped medical schools in Addis Ababa and Salisbury, and later took up permanent appointments in Hong Kong and then Tasmania. Because I was also a career anatomist (rather than a young surgeon working for higher surgical qualifications), I was given his special student teaching task after he left Birmingham.

Teaching and Learning With 'Different' Students

In my first year of this option, I had several mature students, several students with unusual prior preparations (one already a PhD, another a nurse) and, especially, several overseas students. I particularly remember Paul Leung and Buddy Wong from Southeast Asia. (Years later I was to meet father Wong and other Wong brothers in Hong Kong). Tony Waldron was unusual in already having a PhD in lead poisoning. Christine, a qualified nurse, had decided to change careers to do medicine (very unusual in those days). As a result of all this, I gained experience, almost from the beginning, in helping students with unusual backgrounds, many from overseas.

This was furthered when I moved to the University of Chicago where I had, among others, an MD/PhD student named Harry Yang (of Chinese ethnicity but completely American in his upbringing in downstate Illinois). He performed brilliantly in both his MD and his PhD (the latter he did with me, using optical Fourier transforms to examine the internal bony structure in the spines of apes, see elsewhere). He later became a top surgeon in Chicago.

Harry was followed by Artyan Hsu, a Vietnamese doctoral student in physical therapy at the University of Southern California. His English was not very good when I first knew him, but his speaking of mathematics was superb! He worked with me using finite element analysis to study the mechanics of bone form, this time on radiographs of the spongy bone in the human heel in relation to walking (again see elsewhere).

But my main Asian contacts came later to be directly with China, and followed as a result of being invited to be external examiner for Professor Lisowski's medical classes, after he had moved as Head of Department to the University of Hong Kong. Hong Kong only funded me for one year in every three as examiner, but because Peter and I were carrying out research together, and also because I had ample research funding, I was able to visit almost every year until Peter's retirement.

In particular, through Peter's connections with the China Medical Board, there was a period when I was invited to China every second year as a guest of the Chinese Anatomical Society. Their meetings were usually held at one or other of the Sacred Mountains. I especially remember Omei San and Lu San. We also visited, of course, different medical schools, anthropological museums, primate centers and the sites of various fossil finds. These included the Kunming Medical College, the Kunming Primate Research Center, Yuan Mou (the site of the discovery of 'Yuan Mou Man') and Xi'an (with the famous Terracotta Warriors).

It was during this period that I came to know Woo Ju Kang (Wu Rukang) at the Academia Sinica. He was a delightful colleague and we wrote several papers together (including papers in *Nature* based on my statistical analyses of his measurements of the teeth of more than a thousand fossils, see another chapter).

In addition, this period included publishing two books (Figure 12.1) by the University of Hong Kong Press with Kenneth Toogood, Head of the Press at that time. The first book, *The Order of Man*, figured as a frontispiece a painting of a Chinese golden monkey with the title, 'No Tiger in the Mountains', as a part of a little saying that goes:

'No fish in the river, the crab is king,

No tiger in the mountains, the monkey is king'

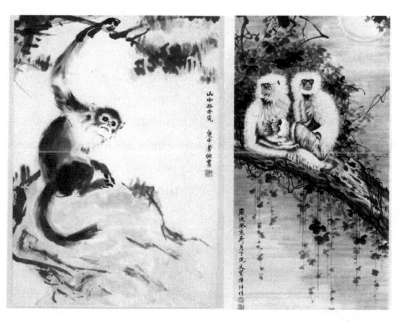

Figure 12.1:   Paintings used as the frontispieces for the two books.

The second book, *Fossils, Teeth and Sex*, figured a Chinese painting of two gibbons with a moon both above and reflected in a pool below, a classical Chinese (and also classical Japanese) artistic theme.

Pan Ruliang: And a Further China-Australia Link

The China connection was continued around 1989 when I started work with Pan Ruliang in Western Australia. I had first met him in Kunming on one of my earlier visits while he was working with Dr. (now Professor) Nina Jablonski. After she moved from Hong Kong to us in Western Australia, he followed her as her doctoral student. Of course, although Pan was young, he was already a fairly senior academic in China with quite a number of publications. But he felt that he needed an understanding of Western science, and that could be best achieved by work with Nina. A little later, Nina left Australia for her home country, the USA, and I became Pan's sole doctoral supervisor.

What was Pan's special need? It was to learn to apply Western scientific methods to his studies of Chinese primates.

I set up a series of meetings with him to discuss what 'Western science' was! He had difficulty framing research questions and criticizing the literature. It was only when I got him to translate one of his own papers that I realized the problem. His papers consisted of:

a statement of his (prior) supervisor's work,
a description of the work he himself had done, and
a conclusion that his results confirmed his supervisor's work!

Though there was much new data, there were no elements of critique, no testing of old ideas and, therefore, no new ideas and no new tests!

I gave him some papers to read and assess, and we had tutorial discussions, but he still had difficulty with criticism.

Finally, in exasperation, I gave him one of my own papers to criticize (it was a paper with a flaw in it). Could he find the flaw? "I cannot do it", he said,

"you are my supervisor!"

It was only then that I understood the problem, and only then that he started to see how important it is to be able to criticize,

not only *others* (that's often quite easy),
not only *colleagues* (more difficult),
but also your *supervisor (mentor)* (this was so difficult for him) and *your own* work (most difficult of all); *your own* thoughts!

These were the methods of Western science that, at that point, were alien to him. Yet he had the insight to know why he wanted to be in Australia.

This all eventually worked out. Pan and I initially worked together, but more importantly, Pan himself, with a little help from me, has become a major researcher.

Pan had other demons to fight. For his doctorate, I was able to fund him as a PhD student from my research grants.

But the next step was postdoctoral funding. We have both never forgotten the time when he was trying to get an Australian Research Council Postdoctoral Research Fellowship. In those days, the candidate's proposed program was assessed numerically. He obtained 97 points out of 100, and as I knew the cut-off for funding was about 80, we were both very pleased. But when the official results came out, he was not on the list.

He was so upset, and I was dumbfounded. I made a private phone call to find out what had happened. My informant was so embarrassed to tell me that Pan's rating, as a foreigner, had been reduced from 97 to 80!

Never mind, I told Pan, we'll try again in the next round. And next time, as a permanent resident, he indeed got it. Subsequently, he and I together had a whole series of Australian Research Council grants.

But this was not the only time he had problems of this sort. I later supported him strongly for a position with tenure at Cape Town. He got it; we were delighted.

Then the terms of appointment were quickly changed! The government decreed that foreigners could not hold tenured positions. His tenure, so hard won, was removed (so much for the meaning of the word 'tenure')! His wife also had a job which, as a foreigner, she also lost. Though Pan was a highly successful researcher and teacher of medical students in South Africa, he was forced eventually to return to Australia. Such a move takes time!

With Pan as the primary investigator, we continued to work on a variety of projects. One set of studies examined the anatomies (largely of the skull) of various species of living Old World monkeys. We found statistical separations that related to sex differences (degrees of dimorphism), functional differences (such as different ways of chewing) and developmental differences (in various skull parts). Our findings were especially strong because of double parallel comparisons that we could make between African and Asian Cercopitheques, and African and Asian Colobines (see other chapters).

Pan's most recent work, however, has stemmed from his worries about what is happening to the environment and ecology.

China: Animal Losses Over Millions of Years

Pan studied Chinese fossils over the last 3 million years. Figures 12.2 to 12.5 each show species losses. *Gigantopithecus* was gone by 1.0

million years, fossil orang utans by 0.7 million years, fossil gibbons by 0.12 million years, and fossil macaques are gone today.

These losses were largely due to tectonic movements, long climactic changes and other natural factors over millions of years.

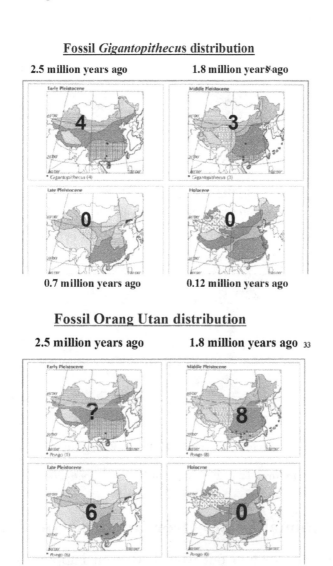

Fossil *Gigantopithecus* distribution

2.5 million years ago   1.8 million years ago

0.7 million years ago   0.12 million years ago

Fossil Orang Utan distribution

2.5 million years ago   1.8 million years ago [33]

0.7 million years ago   0.12 million years ago

Figures 12.2, 12.3, 12.4 and 12.5: Fossil specimens found in China.

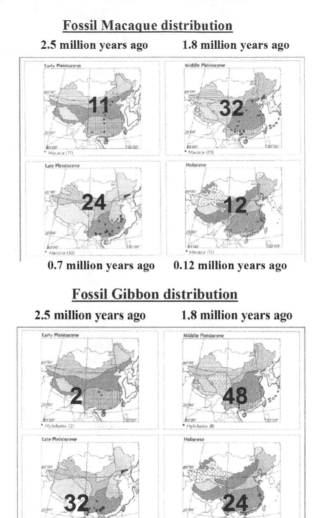

Figures 12.2, 12.3, 12.4 and 12.5:   (*Continued*)

China: Animal Losses Over Hundreds of Years

Pan then tried to find out what had been happening over the last 600 years. He could do this by examining the records of the Cantons (Figure 12.6).

**Records of Cantons about animals caught for food are
so good that Pan Ruliang (who of course can read
Chinese) could identify them down to species**

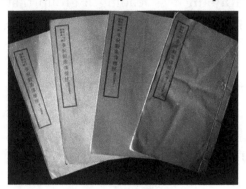

Figure 12.6: Records of the Cantons.

The descriptions of the animals are so good that Pan could identify them down to the species level. Figures 12.7, 12.8 and 12.9 show reductions of golden monkeys from 11 provinces 400 years ago to 7 provinces 200 years ago, to only 3 provinces, 50 years ago. These reductions are largely due to community needs for food and medicines!

China: Animal Losses Today

This naturally led Pan to examine more recent times. These are mainly related to societal, industrial, economic and political changes in China's development (Figure 12.10).

The evidence of today's problems can be seen by trawling through Google (Figures 12.11 to 12.21)!

Problems for animal species today are evident in Figures 12.15 to 12.21.

All this work, led by Pan Ruliang, and involving many Chinese and International colleagues still goes on. I am honoured to be included in some of it.

China and the World: Hoping for the Future

By 2016, **Pan Ruliang** was leading a group that included four Chinese collaborators (Li B., Qi X., He G. and Guo S.), an American

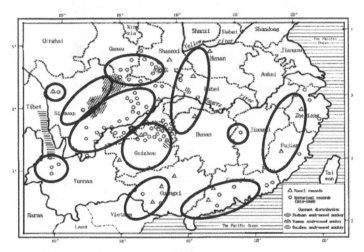

Golden monkeys in 11 Provinces 400 years ago

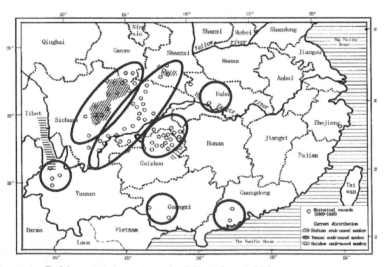

Golden monkeys in only 7 Provinces 200 years ago

Figures 12.7, 12.8 and 12.9:   Changes in numbers of golden monkey species in Chinese provinces over time.

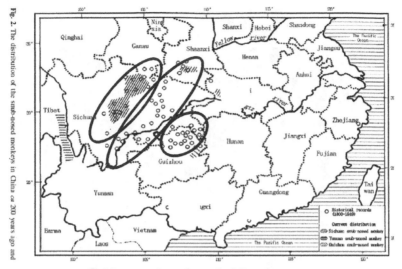

Fig. 2. The distribution of the snub-nosed monkeys in China ca 200 years ago and

Golden monkeys in only 3 Provinces now

Figures 12.7, 12.8 and 12.9: *(Continued)*

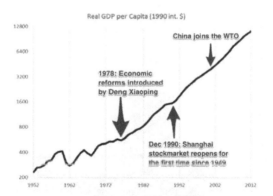

Hirst T. 2015 (A brief history of China's economic growth)

Figure 12.10: China's economic growth in recent years.

(Paul Garber), and his Australian Colleagues (Cyril Grueter and I). We published:

'A new conservation strategy for China: a model starting with Primates' in the *American Journal of Primatology*.

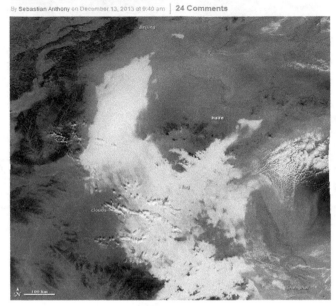

Fig. 12.11:   Evidence of pollution over most of China.

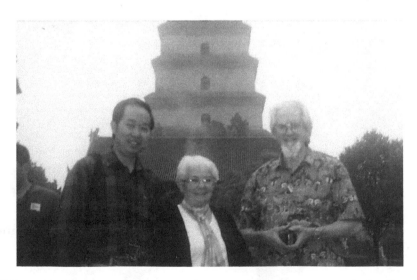

Fig. 12.12:   Pan, my wife Eleanor, and me. It's not a bad picture; just bad pollution.

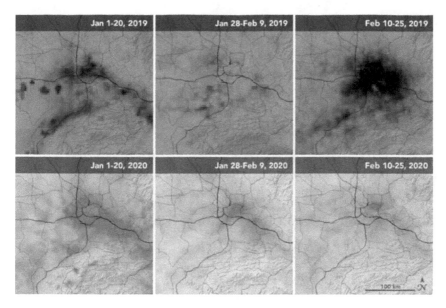

Figure 12.13: Change over a year! Pollution in 2019 in Hubei compared with 2020 in which the coronavirus pandemic and lockdown had occurred.

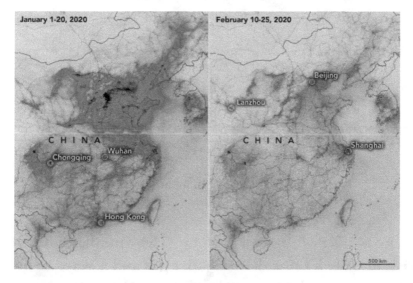

Figure 12.14: The situation in the whole of China: the effect of one month of industrial shutdown as a result of the coronavirus!

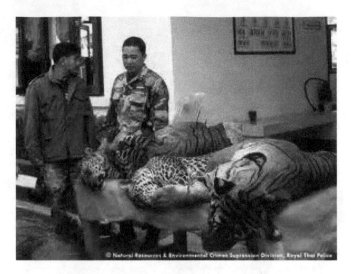

Figure 12.15:   Problems for big cats in China.

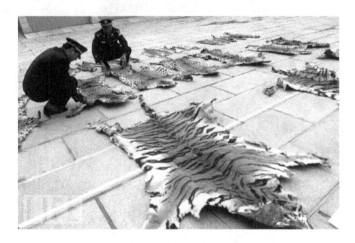

Figure 12.16:   Problems for tigers in China.

In 2018, this was followed by **'The Animal Extinction Crisis in China: Immediate Challenges and a Way Forward'** in *Biodiversity and Conservation*, Springer, Nature BV.

At this point **Pan** was leading an expanded group of workers: 13 Chinese, 3 Australians, 2 Brazilians, 1 Mexican and 1 American.

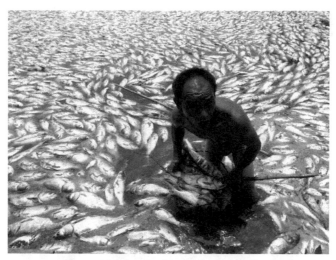

Figure 12.17: Problems for fish in China.

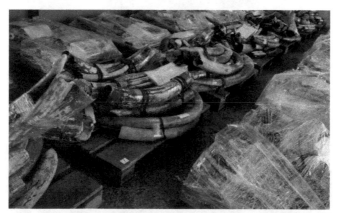

Figure 12.18: Problems for elephants in China.

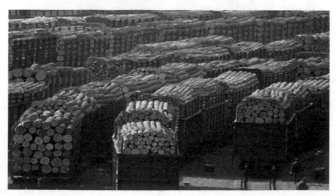

Figure 12.19: Problems for trees in China.

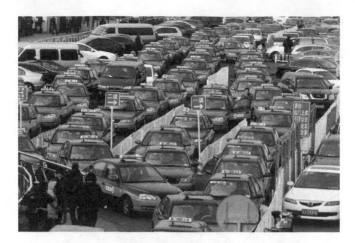

Figure 12.20:   Problems for people in China.

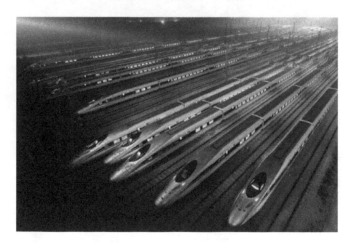

Figure 12.21:   Yet other problems in China today. Cost of this rail system: more than $30 billion (within China's total research and development of more than $2 trillion).

(It is sad to record that one of our colleagues, Professor Colin Groves from the Australian National University, has since died.)

In 2019, **Pan** and eight other Chinese colleagues, using drone technology, published a truly modern investigation titled '**Using Unmanned Aerial Vehicles with Thermal-Image Acquisition Cameras for Animal Surveys: A Case Study of the Sichuan**

Snub-Nosed Monkey in the Qinling Mountains' (authors: Haitao Yang, **Ruliang Pan**, Yewen Sun, Pengbin Zheng, Jinghua Wang, Xuelin Jin, Jingjie Zhang, Baogou Li and Songtao Guo) in *Integrative Zoology*.

In 2020, Pan and eight others published '**Macaques in China: Evolutionary Dispersion and Subsequent Development'** (authors: Baoguo Li, Gang He, Songtao Guo, Rong Hou, Kang Huang, Pei Zhang, He Zhang, **Ruliang Pan** and Colin A. Chapman) in the *American Journal of Primatology*.

And in this current year, Pan and I are involved in a submission entitled '**The Impending Extinction of Non-Human Primates in East Asia'** (authors: Baoguo Li, He Zhang, Jiqi, Lu, Shiyi Tang, Zhipang Huang, Liangwei Cui, Daoying Lan, Rong Hou, Wen Xiao, Songtao Guo, Gang He, Kang Huang, Pei Zhang, Hao Pan, **Charles Oxnard** and **Ruliang Pan**).

All these ideas, in the face of global climate change, increasing habitat degradation, deforestation, pollution of air, earth and water (largely industrial), and an impending worldwide animal and plant extinction crisis, has lead **Pan** to convene a group of internationally distinguished, concerned and conservation-oriented scientists and conservationists to come together as the **International Centre of Biodiversity and Primate Conservation** (ICBPC).

The ICBPC is housed at Dali University, Yunnan Province, China. It operates through Dali and Northwest Universities, two distinguished educational institutions in China, and has a highly respected board of international conservation scientists and experts, donors, environmental journalists, entrepreneurs and political leaders. All are dedicated to protecting the world's environment. I am privileged to have been appointed (2020) as Honorary Executive Committee Member of the Board.

The ICBPC aims to share the combined experience and expertise of these international experts in conservation biology, genetics, animal behavior, community ecology, disease and ecosystem health, and environmental sustainability. The aim is to work with local and regional scientists, conservation organizations, governmental officials, the media, educators and the public to help preserve, protect and restore natural habitats and threatened animals and plants.

To accomplish this, the group is compiling regional and national archives of environmental information as an integrated repository for data management, data analysis, computer modelling, wildlife videos and the implementation of sustainable conservation policies and actions (to promote biodiversity, habitat restoration and public education). It aims to describe the most recent advances in climate science, sustainable land use patterns, animal and plant species requirements, good governance and the needs of the local human communities that overlap with animal and plant distributions.

The ICBPC is located in southwestern China, a region of great animal and plant biodiversity that covers Yunnan and Tibet, and is home to more than 26 human cultural and ethnic groups as well as more than 15 nonhuman primate species. It contains also several World Heritage Sites, most notably the 'Three Parallel Rivers' (Yangtze, Mekong and Salween). It is a global 'hotspot' that includes high plateaus, tropical and subtropical forests, evergreen and deciduous broad-leafed forests, coniferous forests and alpine shrubs and meadows. The three major rivers make unique contributions to the biological diversity of 15,000 plant species, 250 species of mammals and 780 species of birds.

The initial focus of the ICBPC's activities is China. Results described above already show that China is facing an unprecedented set of challenges in balancing the effects of economic development and global climate change with environmental protection and maintaining biodiversity. China is the world's most populous nation, and has transitioned from a largely agrarian to a highly industrial economy over the past 50 years. The effect of this has been to transform its natural environment in ways that have negatively impacted the environment and species survival. Across China, there is very limited public awareness of the impending animal (and for that matter too, plant) extinction crisis.

Therefore, the ICBPC plans to promote interdisciplinary research between Chinese and international experts. The hope is to work collaboratively with large and varied data sets to develop strategies, policies and management tools, in conjunction with local governments, business leaders, NGOs and global citizens, to conserve and protect living things and their environments.

Pan has been pursuing these ideas for a long time. However, in addition to persuading the people of the world to realize the danger of life extinctions, we also have to fight the growing tribalisms and nationalisms that are resisting these global actions!

This **China connection**, and especially the initial collaboration and friendship with **Wu Rukang** (in earlier times) and the work and friendship with **Pan Ruliang** (today), has been amongst the most challenging, but also the most satisfying, of my scientific life.

Part 4

Challenging Inside the Ivory Tower

Chapters 13–17

Student rebellions are nothing new today. But they were unusual at the time, particularly before the Vietnam War when I was still a student. The few rebellions that occurred were usually about trying to improve things for students. It would have been most out of character for me to have been involved; I was the epitome of the student 'swot'.

Yet by accident, from my earliest undergraduate days, I have found myself trying to change, sequentially, students, universities, medical schools, hospitals and, eventually and even more widely, education and society! Such changing recognizes that research, teaching and practice are not the only activities we should undertake. Every bit as important is challenging the systems within which we work. Goodness knows, they need change.

Of course, most of us hold almost unquestioning loyalty to the educational systems within which we have been brought up, and it is right that we should. Such loyalty for me started with being a student in a grammar school founded in 1614! And it continued for me as a physician through the Convention of Geneva (based on the older Hippocratic Oath) that we duly signed at medical graduation: "I will give to my teachers the respect and gratitude which is their due."

Yet loyalty must always be seasoned. It cannot
be blind loyalty!

We must learn how to challenge especially our institutions. They aren't always right. Can this lead to hope? Hope that our institutions improve, rather than get worse! I wonder if the lessons I learnt as a student rebel would still be operative today.

In my student days, we had the feeling that we students were important. It is true we were only small parts of an institution: a university, of a discipline: science, of a profession: medicine, and of a society: both national and international. To all of these we had loyalties, and to all we were expected to contribute. Of course, we knew that we were at the bottom of the pile. In science and medicine, professors and consultants were at the top! This was certainly true in England when I graduated.

How different it is today. Professors are often at the bottom; administrators and government are always at the top. You students have a curious, intermediate, yet floating position because you carry much of the money to them. You have more clout than professors. Certainly, the university administration is more afraid of you students than professors!

Chapter 13: Students Effecting Change; <u>Is</u> it Possible?

An Undergraduate Student Challenging the University!   364

Chapter 14: Professors Effecting Change; It is Impossible!

Chapter 15: Deans Effecting Change; The Poisoned Chalice: Is it Ever Possible?

Chapter 16: The Conscience of the University!

Chapter 17: Military Interludes!

Chapter 13

Students Effecting Change; Is It Possible?

My student challenging started like this. As a third-year undergraduate, I was elected as Chairman of the Athletic Union, the overarching organization for sports at the university. Usually the Chairman held office for only a single year because he (in those days it was always a man!) was usually elected in his final year. But as a medical student in a six-year curriculum, it turned out that I would come to hold office for three years; this was unique.

Usually, too, the Chairman of the Athletic Union (i.e., of all sports clubs) was also captain of one of the major sports teams: soccer, rugby, hockey, et cetera, and this left little time for him to do much with the Athletic Union; he was typically too busy with his Autumn and Spring team sport. But because I was captain of athletics, which in England operates only in the summer term, I had spare time in the first two terms.

Usually there were no really major matters to be sorted out by the Athletic Union. The individual sports clubs largely ran themselves; the Athletic Union merely awarded 'blues' to the top performers and apportioned the budget among the different sports clubs. Someone had to do it!

Therefore, in my free time in those first two terms, I started to survey all the sports facilities in the university and, more importantly, compare them with equivalent facilities at similar 'red brick' universities in England. (I was using the scientific method that I had just learnt during my BSc honors research year.)

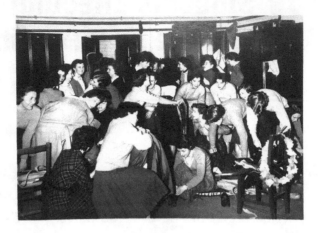

Figure 13.1:   Part of the evidence: I was allowed to take a photo in the heavily crowded women's changing room. The woman in the dark dress lower left was the women's hockey captain, Ann Ballantyne, now Dr. Ann Fawcett, then my Athletic Union Vice-Chair!

I received enormous help in this survey. The Athletic Union Permanent Secretary (a very gracious lady) agreed to type everything, and as we ended up with a 22-page document going through several drafts, that was a lot of work. The Medical School Librarian (my librarian girlfriend's supervisor, who therefore also liked me), also helped. She contacted her librarian friends in other universities. Can you imagine university librarians all over the country measuring changing rooms, counting showers, baths and loos, estimating student usage, even counting outdoor sports pitches? I developed a 'comparative anatomy' of our sports facilities. We did not look good (Figure 13.1).

An Undergraduate Student Challenging the University!

Then, from out of the blue, a wonderful thing happened: **The Vice-Chancellor intervened**.

The Vice-Chancellor of the University (Sir Robert Aitken) wrote to the Chairman of the Athletic Union (me) pointing out that the university was squeezed for building space, and that the students would have to give up the sports fields (rugby, soccer, hockey) that graced the front of the university campus. He was truly sorry about this, he said, but noted that the university's Planning and Priorities Committee were looking toward installing some new indoor sports facilities (table tennis, squash, etc) including an indoor swimming pool which, he said, he was aware that the students badly wanted. He expressed the hope that the students would be willing to give up the outside sports fields with the provision of these new inside facilities. He needed my reaction quickly.

Until the moment I received that letter, **I did not know** that changing the sports facilities was **in train**.

However, when he sent that letter, **he did not know** that, totally by accident, my sports facilities survey was also **in train** (and in fact, **almost finished**).

The result was that, within two weeks, I was able to place the 22-page report on his desk. It described the parlous state of our sports facilities compared with other universities. Further, aided by David Munrow, the Head of Physical Education, I was also able to provide the VC with an appendix of a list of needs. It was a carefully reasoned set of requests.

However, in the very last line of the report, I wrote:

"I feel sure that the students will not be bribed into giving up playing fields by the provision of a swimming pool."

Within thirty minutes of that report landing on his desk, I was summoned to the VC's office. For about thirty minutes, apparently in a most irritated manner, he dressed me up hill and down dale. Then, I remember it so clearly, a twinkle came to his eye.

"If you are willing to remove the word 'bribed' from the last sentence, I'll take it to Planning and Priorities."

Of course, I did. And he did.

The upshot was that the Planning and Priorities Committee accepted our report and planned a 125 acre (as I remember it) playing field site at Wast Hills away from the University. The small hills on the site were not suitable for playing fields, but the remainder of the site provided some 60 acres that were overlooked by the hills, a beautiful location.

It took about a further two years for this to actually happen. But happen it did, and as a three-year Chairman of the Athletic Union, I was still there to see it. We were overjoyed! And Sir Robert was a wonderful example of someone capable of changing his mind based on evidence.

There is an appendix to this story. Even now, more than 50 years later, our beautiful playing fields at the entrance to the university have still not been built on. A double win!

This success generated a request from the medical students at Queens Medical Society, who asked me to prepare a case for improved medical student facilities, lounge rooms, canteens, locker rooms, and so on, to the Faculty of Medicine.

A Medical Student Challenging the Medical School

Hence, I did a somewhat similar thing; I surveyed equivalent facilities at comparable medical schools and prepared a report. Again, compared to other schools, we did not look good. I used the word 'bribed' again, with a similar result! That report, and the seminar based on it that I gave to the medical faculty, won me the Richard's Memorial Prize that year.

However, far more importantly, the Dean of Medicine was converted. New facilities were planned and provided. Because a new medical library was being built, the old library premises were altered to become a student facility. Of course, this was a long time ago; there have been several further sets of improvements in the medical student facilities over the years. I would scarcely recognize the student facilities there today.

One might get the impression that I was a student rebel. In fact, that was not so. My time was a few years before the student rebellions. I 'rebelled' by being 'reasonable' (except for that word 'bribed'), by being a little 'crafty' (I always 'lobbied' the professors on the relevant committees), and especially by applying the 'comparative method' that I had learnt in my research year (no one wants to be seen as 'bested')!

Then, almost by accident, I took a third rebellious step.

A 'Young Doctor' Challenging the Hospital!

The term 'young doctor' was the euphemism employed by the hospital when it introduced us students to patients, nurses, 'real' doctors and other staff. **They all knew we weren't real!**

The time came when, naturally, I had a run-in with the hospital administration. It involved my time in obstetrics.

In those days, obstetrics was done 'on the district'. When called, often in the middle of the night, we would go out with our little black bag into the slums of Birmingham to 'deliver' babies. The little black bag was our passport to some of the rougher areas in town. With that bag, we could go anywhere and were helped by all the locals.

Well, I said to deliver babies, because what we did was called a delivery, but in the beginning, we mainly just watched while the far more experienced midwives did the delivery. Later we were allowed to assist said midwives, and once they trusted us, we delivered the babies ourselves. The midwives would nevertheless be staring over our shoulders, ready to tear our hands away if they saw us doing something wrong!

In any case, 'delivery' often involved doing the opposite: 'BBB', or *beating baby back*, so as to prevent the baby from emerging too quickly and causing a perineal tissue tear. And if we were unable to prevent a tear or if we had to do an episiotomy, we had to sew it up ourselves. We all learnt.

As an aside, I have never forgotten a student colleague who was attending a delivery on the district. He had arrived late, after the birth; this often happened! The birth had already been conducted by an old crone. When he got there, the baby had been washed, the mother had her cup of tea, but — and it was a very large but — **the placenta was sizzling and burning on the fire!**

It was therefore not possible for him to examine the placenta to check that it was all there. We were supposed to cup it in our hands to see if, perhaps, one of the bits of cotyledons was missing. A cotyledon retained in the uterus is a serious matter, requiring in those days admission to hospital, treatment with an antibiotic and removal under an anesthetic. But my friend could not retrieve the placenta from the fire to check! So, he had to call the consultant, who was a bit annoyed with the situation but knew that the mother had to be admitted just in case.

However, returning to my main story, it was just my luck. At the time when I expected to do my obstetrics, the system was changed. Henceforth obstetric clerks in the professorial unit were to deliver babies in the internal obstetric unit of the Queen Elizabeth Hospital.

The General Medical Council's requirement (not the medical school's) was that we had to deliver and, more importantly, be signed up for twenty normal births. But now that we were working in the hospital milieu, we had to compete for normal births with the pupil midwives. As they were only allowed normal deliveries, it was quite a fight for a medical student in a hospital to get twenty 'normals'! Many hospital births were not 'normal'. However, we also participated in the abnormal births in which the pupil midwives were not involved. So, we got extra experience that we would never have obtained 'on the district'.

Some of these 'abnormal' cases were so sad, but also so important, for the training of doctors in those days. He (it was almost always a he), on qualification, might find himself drafted into the armed services as a doctor; might find himself in somewhere like Malaya (as it was then); might perhaps be the only doctor for not only for his unit but also thousands of local civilians without any other doctor. So, in those days he had to be able to deliver babies, handle simple obstetric complications, perform appendectomies 'on the kitchen table', handle less serious trauma, and so on, even just soon after full registration.

'Fighting' with the pupil midwives for 'normal' cases also gave us a real idea of how hard they had to work. Peculiarly enough, it generated an understanding and good relations among us. More than one of us later married 'ex-pupil midwives'! So, it was all good.

Of course, we had to live in the new system because we could be called at any time of the day or night. So, we were provided with a bedroom.

But when the four of us arrived that first day, we realized that, unusually (for those days), we comprised three women and myself! We went to see the administration to get another room; men and women did not — and absolutely could not — sleep together in those days. At least not as sanctioned by the administration! Yes, we'll fix it, they said. But four o'clock came, they all went home, and it was not fixed.

We decided that we knew how to fix it. I would sleep with the women! *Which I did! If only I could remember who they were?*

Rather to our surprise, no one took a blind bit of notice. The next day: still no room! We conferred and decided that we should get it fixed somehow.

So, I slept in the labor ward on the second night, and it was quite a disturbed night.

But again, no one seemed in the slightest bit bothered. The patients and nurses in the delivery room were too busy to take any notice of me!

I then applied my newly developed administrative skills and took matters into my own hands. I took my bed and rolled it into the Professor's Office (Professor Hugh McLaren: years later he was to deliver our two boys). There must have been no babies that night. I was still asleep in his office when he came in the next morning.

We had an extra room that very day; a challenging success!

Challenging the Very Pinnacle: The Court of Governors

My last student rebellion came when, as a final year medical student, I was elected for a five-year term to the Court of Governors of the University of Birmingham. The part I would play in the university's governance was very small. I was one of only three students on that very large body; one of three, among many dozens of other categories!

The Court of Governors only met once a year. The President and Vice President of the Guild of Undergraduates were always members *ex officio*; the third position usually went to the Guild Secretary. But the third position was, technically, a matter of student election, although there never had been an election until my time! And that third position was for five years; therefore, for me, four of those years were while I was past student status!

I decided to stand, and I won. The student who was the Guild Secretary was very upset! And the university administration was somewhat worried. They wanted to know, was Oxnard going to cause trouble at the annual Court of Governors meeting? Of course, in such a large and august body, I had almost no voice. But I enjoyed the meetings each year and met many people.

Student Challenges Many Years Later

Yet another link with student challenges occurred many years later at the University of Chicago (as outlined elsewhere) during the time of the student troubles. Students were involved in protests about many things: the Vietnam war, the military draft (burning draft cards for example), science for the people, the black panthers, and so on. Because I was travelling back and forth to the UK for research collaborations, I just happened to see the different ways that student protests occurred in the two countries. In the US, we had students who were killed by the police on the campus of Kent State University. We had a faculty member have his hand almost severed at the University of Chicago. Someone was killed at the University of Wisconsin, and so on.

On my way to lunch one day in Chicago, I was animatedly discussing science with a colleague and didn't see a line of students standing there with their arms held out. I ran into a student's fist. I was so shocked that *if I had had a gun, I would have shot him.* Perhaps this shows how bad reactions can occur!

Those student troubles culminated in a student sit-down in the administration building. The students hoped to be able to close the university.

The treatment for this condition was usually for the president of the university to call in the police, as indeed had happened at Kent State University.

But our President, Edward Levi, was cleverer than that. He did not call in the police. Indeed, he did nothing, because something the students did not realize was that most of the U of C administrators were academics providing administrative services part-time. When they were denied access to the administration building, they just carried on their administration in their academic offices and laboratories. So, the university continued to run without hindrance.

The students sat-in. But gradually the numbers sitting-in fell and fell until, about two weeks later, the last of them left with their tails between their legs as it were. At this point, Edward had the building opened for everyone in the neighborhood to see the damage they had done (e.g., excrement stuffed in the typewriters and smeared on the walls). But importantly, no armed police were involved, and no one was killed!

It was therefore of great interest to me to see how these US cases compared with what happened at the University of Birmingham, UK. I just happened to be back in Birmingham for research purposes at the time when the students there decided to have a sit-in. About fifty students 'sat in' the university's Great Hall. They were not causing any disruption to the university because that space was only used for convocations and so on. But the then Birmingham Vice-Chancellor called in the police!

The student reaction: immediately, the fifty or so students swelled to about five hundred.

The police reaction: when the police came, they had no guns; it was England! And the 'police' consisted only of one long, thin constable and one large, fat sergeant. They walked into the middle of the student mob, and the fat sergeant told the constable what to say. With his bullhorn, the constable warned:

"You are all committing a trespass. Will you please leave?"

Such is the power of the English Bobby at that time, and perhaps also the power of the biblical and legal word 'trespass', that the students all quietly got up and left.

Wonderful differences between two societies and among three universities! And wonderful aims for students!

14 Professors Effecting Change; It <u>Is</u> Impossible!

My first entrée into administration as a professor was in Chicago, and it involved the medical curriculum. Of course, curriculum is always a contentious issue, and never more so than in medicine. *There are so many oxen to be gored!*

The Medical Student Curriculum

The medical school had set up a curriculum committee to consider change in the medical curriculum. As a new professor (this was just after my move to the USA), I had not had time to make any enemies. Also, I didn't know anything about the US curriculum, plus I had no experience of the American system. So, naturally, it was decreed that I would not only be a member, but the chairman!

I pondered for a while on how to get the discussion going. Obviously, we needed information, so yet again I did a survey — precisely the tactic that I had used as a student in the UK! As a result, I thought the problems were obvious. But I had to work out how to set up the discussion without everyone being up in arms. So, I got the committee to first discuss curriculum at a dinner.

I arranged it so that there was a single long table. Down the length of the table I had a double centerpiece: two rolls of white wallpaper. On those rolls, in topic groups, I stuck down the title of every lecture, every tutorial, every seminar and every lab. But I arranged them in subject blocks without attributing any of them to any particular department.

People arrived, and even before the soup came, they were reading the lists. They were even changing positions at the table so that they could read the whole thing. There was considerable silence while this was going on.

There were **some 70-plus class titles on DNA, RNA and related matters** at one part of the centerpiece! These titles did not involve much repetition, each department teaching its own brand.

Another part of the centerpiece contained **about 30 titles covering carbohydrate metabolism and related information**. Again, little true repetition; each department covering its own parts.

In splendid isolation was **the heart: one lecture!** Yet heart disease is the greatest of killers.

Discussion started. For the first time, I saw little 'needle' between departments. The imbalance was so obvious; the numbers made it clear that something had to be done. And so, indeed, we got a new curriculum quite quickly.

Of course, there was one special feature that made this process easier at Chicago than at most other universities. Departmental funding at Chicago did not depend upon student numbers! No given unit was fighting for dollars, for 'bums on *their* seats'!

The Medical Student Intake

A little later I was placed on another committee to discuss increasing the medical student intake (amazing how new staff are slated for these kinds of committees!). Student admissions were carried out, absolutely admirably, by Professor Joe Ceithaml, Dean of Students. Yet even he, with his vast experience, was feeling pressures, hence the committee.

We used to have approximately 6,000 applicants, as I remember it, for 98 places. Of course, this very large number was because of multiple applications by each hopeful student. In England at that time, in contrast, students usually only applied to a small number of medical schools; I myself applied to only one!

Winnowing 6,000 applicants for 98 places is a bit silly. Any random 98 from only the top 1,000 would probably have given a class no better or worse than any other random class from the top 1,000, however selected. Normally, student admissions handled it. The 6,000 were rapidly boiled down to the top 1,000, then winnowed to 300, and only the top among the 300 were interviewed by academic staff. This was a complex and longwinded process. Inevitably, however, the classes were very good.

The task of this new committee was to discuss increasing the size of the medical class. The government had decreed that we needed more doctors.

In contradistinction to the abovementioned curriculum committee, this one sat for almost two years! It eventually came up with its recommendation.
To increase the size of the class from 98 to 102!
An elephant giving birth to a mouse!

It reminded me of All Souls College which, in my time in the UK, had no undergraduates at all. A British governmental review suggested that they should take undergraduates. The College solemnly agreed; *it decided to take one!* One very lucky person!

Medical Titles

Yet another committee on which I served involved designing new titles for medical clinicians at a hospital in downtown Chicago. An agreement had been struck to include this hospital in the group of hospitals serving our medical school. I was the person (the youngest, newest!) designated to take notes of all discussions and to prepare minutes to help get a report going.

This was a very high-level committee and it was a very important task; the question of titles always raises much concern. And, it seems, even more concern in medicine than in any other area!

As a result, I came to know some of the top people in the university. I believe it was my usefulness to this committee that drew me to the attention of the President who later offered me the Deanship of the College (of Letters, Arts and Sciences).

Dean of Letters, Arts and Sciences

Even this was an interesting task. The Dean of each of the graduate divisions of the university would be chosen from among the major professors in each specific division. The major professors were largely from abroad; I seem to remember that about 70% of the faculty had overseas qualifications. And my remembery also is that only about 20% of the students came from Chicago and Illinois. Most students were from out of state, and quite a number, indeed, from out of country.

Thus, in addition to me (British) being Dean of the College, the Dean of Law was Australian, the Dean of Physical Sciences was also Australian and was later followed by an Indian, the Dean of Divinity was Jewish and was followed later by a Japanese, and the Dean of Humanities was Dutch (who had spent a considerable portion of his life hiding inside the walls of a house in Holland whenever the Gestapo came around) and was later followed by a Jew. Any scrutiny of Chicago's many Nobel Prize winners over the years indicates just how worldwide the faculty were! There was generally no problem.

But the Deanship of the college was different. The college was an amalgam of biological, physical, social, and humanities collegiate divisions, together with a fifth called, for want of a better name, the New Collegiate Division. The idea of this college was the academic descendant of the 'Hutchins College' of an earlier time. In contrast to the Deans of the graduate divisions, the College Dean was almost always an inside appointment, and had usually been chosen in rotation from the different collegiate divisions.

At this point, it was biology's turn. But for internal political reasons, it was not easy to choose anyone from the biology collegiate division. Edward Levi cut the Gordian Knot. I, of course, was not in the college, I was in the biological sciences graduate division (and the medical school which was a subunit of biological sciences — itself an interesting relationship!). Edward realized that though I was a physician and in the medical school, I also had degrees in biological and bioengineering sciences. What better way to appoint, as the new College Dean, a biologist who, though from the university (i.e., internal), was not from the college. I was therefore without the baggage that the various college possibilities carried at that time.

A typical Chicago solution, and a fascinating opportunity for me.

Most individuals are loyal to the education they received. I was no different, *until I got to Chicago*. Then I changed; I started to recognize that, though I got my degrees in the UK, I was being educated at the University of Chicago!

As the College Dean, I completely accepted the changeover from the narrowing down of the traditional British undergraduate curriculum to the broadening up (the liberal arts) of the Chicago college (and also Columbia, Annapolis St. Johns, and probably others). Students got a lick of many things. A student could change from one major to another without loss. Every student got their final preferred major, and all students could add ancillaries of their choice. There was no rigid framework; everyone had to be both narrowly and broadly educated!

What then was the problem? It was this: In the earlier years of the Hutchins College, the university had attracted many of the top academics in the US. Hutchins had decreed that these very high-quality research academics were to also provide very high-quality undergraduate teaching. And it worked. The 'Hutchins College' (and a couple of other US institutions, like Columbia and Annapolis St. Johns) became well-known for the excellence of their undergraduate education and the idea of general education. University of Chicago alumni were extremely loyal to the 'Hutchins College'. But that had been many years before.

Times change. Funds reduce. Individuals retire without replacement. The college from being good was having difficulties. It was necessary to do something about it. Thus, the university had been reducing the college staff (by natural retirements and non-replacements), while at the same time trying to increase the numbers of undergraduates. Most of the staff reductions had been carried out in the time of prior College Deans. By the time I was appointed, these reductions had been largely achieved. Only about half-a-dozen of the earlier staff were still there. In theory, there were many vacancies.

How then to attract more good undergraduates and more good teachers? President Levi's answer was to decree that graduate division professors (some of the best investigators in the country in their various disciplines) should teach in the college. However, it was easy for him to decree that, but it was for the Deans of the college to make it happen. The problem was well on the way to being solved by Deans prior to me.

I was left with the last part: how to persuade the last of the older staff to go, and how to persuade more professors (but only those who were good teachers!) from the graduate divisions to teach in the college. By my time, there were only about six of the older individuals left. Instead of pressing for redundancies, I discussed with each one the best ways in which they could now contribute. And I discussed with the Deans of the graduate divisions which of their professors could help in the college. And I pressed for "teaching by involvement in research. It is not too much to hope for!" — a concept I had borrowed from an earlier Dean.

All this worked, and was a major success for President Levi. As a graduate division professor who had almost accidentally became Dean of the undergraduate college, I was happy to do this: a research professor becoming involved in undergraduate teaching and university service.

15

Chapter

Deans Effecting Change; The Poisoned Chalice: Is It <u>Ever</u> Possible?

Some years later, moving on to another institution, the University of Southern California, I served a five-year term as Dean of the graduate school (while also having the title of University Research Professor and maintaining an active research program). Thus I managed to escape the technicalities of research administration. That task was carried out by an administrator who, in any case, knew far more than I did about private, state and federal research-funding bodies. My task was to help further strengthen internal research.

Of course, there were many committees in which, as Graduate Dean, I was involved. One of the most interesting of these related to the tenure and appointments of professors.

Administration as a New Dean: Poisoned Chalice Number One

Thus, as Graduate Dean, I was Chair of the final all-university committee reporting to the President on professorial promotions and appointments.

Promotion to tenured associate and full professorships were complex processes, with committees at departmental, faculty and

■383

all-university levels, and with alternating academic and administrative decisions. No one (in theory) could be denied tenure or promotion until there was a 'turn down' at two consecutive levels.

At that time, I had two parts in this process; first as Dean of the graduate school at the administrative level for the graduate school faculty, and then as Chairman of the all-university committee making the final academic-level recommendations for all staff to the President.

As a new person, I found a maelstrom of a system. Because the matter was 'university-wide', there was faculty representation from many different disciplines on the all-university committee. But to reduce the size of the task, the overall committee was divided into a number of smaller committees. Related academic areas were aggregated. For example, the professional social science-type schools (e.g., law and public administration) were done by the same committee that handled the academic social science-type departments (say, economics and political science).

By going through the records, I discovered that this had occasioned terrible arguments and discussions, and worse, a great deal of dissatisfaction and even anger with the process. The economists on the committee were angry because a law academic might be promoted with just a handful of published works (and many of those in non-academic places). In comparison, economists had to have large numbers of publications in the top peer-reviewed economics journals.

Similarly, there was dissatisfaction with decisions in the science committee because while some biochemists might publish a large number of short papers each year, some biologists might only write a major monograph once every three years.

Another difficult (but most interesting) case was creative writing. This was a very strong group because of the propinquity of Hollywood. However, creative writers do not generally have a PhD. In fact, many of them have no university qualifications at all. Getting them appointed and tenured through this type of committee was like pulling teeth.

In creative writing were two of our most 'creative' individuals, author Christopher Isherwood and his partner, artist Don Bachardy. They were earlier escapees, as homosexuals, from the UK! Eleanor and I especially knew Don Bachardy as he nursed Christopher in his last — and sadly, demented — days. Indeed, we possess a signed sketch of Eleanor (see the frontispiece) by Don (but he never gave us the original!). We also have a remarkable book of Don's works that included, at the end, several sketches of Christopher's body after death, showing the changes that occur in those after-death hours — a remarkably poignant offering.

Two more remarkable people in creative writing were Leon and Marta Furtwanger, pre-war literary escapees from Hitler's Germany. Degrees or no degrees, both were clearly top people! They were a joy to meet. Need I say more?

Yet a committee of professors had great difficulty conferring tenure to such distinguished individuals. Sheeesh!

As a new Dean, I felt that I had to try to fix such problems. As a new person, this might be my best and only chance. This one was easy. By the simple act of taking creative writing into my own area, the graduate school, I was indicating to the rest of the university that I thought creative writing was a very important graduate subject, PhD or no PhD!

Tenure and Promotion: Poisoned Chalice Number Two

Then came the case of the social sciences committee, and of the promotion of lawyers to full professorships. I was very lucky to be able to solve this one with help from Edward Levi who at that point was Attorney General of the United States, but who had been the President of the University of Chicago at the time that I was College Dean there. (Indeed, he it was who appointed me to that position.)

I wrote to Edward asking him if he could let me have the *curricula vitarum* of an *aliquot* of the best academic lawyers in the USA. (There has been so much academic argument about the plural of the word: CV!). Some of the people on the list that he sent me were almost household names (e.g., Phil Kurland, a top constitutional lawyer at the University of Chicago). I went through his list and abstracted career data at the point at which the individuals were promoted.

It turned out that, at the point of tenure, most of them had only a few writings that one might call publications. But the importance of those publications was clear. Sometimes one would consist of a major paper covering a whole area distilled from a number of years of important legal cases. Another would consist of a major brief relating to important matters on the practical side of their legal experience. Many times these were not papers in journals in the general academic sense, but rather works in other legal outlets. This was the general theme for most of these very distinguished people (their subsequent careers being evidence they were truly distinguished!).

As an aside, in much more recent years, I had a distinguished legal colleague (a law school Dean, no less) whose publication in the

Harvard Law Review was severely marked down by his university! The deed was done by an administrator who had noted that the *Harvard Law Review* had students on its editorial board. The administrator therefore assumed that it could not be a strong publication. She did not know that it is, perhaps, the highest ranking legal journal in the English-speaking world. Harvard merely adds to the education of a few of their top law students by involving them in the editing process! This is what can happen when decisions are 'administrative'. This decision could not be corrected; so powerful are today's administrators!

I have my own personal example of this type of administrative interference in assessment. I was invited to be Leverhulme Professor at University College London for a whole year (a very prestigious appointment). My professorial brief was not only to carry out research, but also to give a series of public research lectures. Well and good.

However, the Leverhulme Foundation were willing to allow me to advertise my next research book (principally titled *Ghostly Muscles, Wrinkled Brains, Heresies and Hobbits*) with the subtitle of *A Leverhulme Public Lecture Series*, given that my public lectures were based on the research in that book. At this point, administration came back to bite me. The relevant administrator at the University of Western Australia was unable to see that it was a research book; she saw only the words 'Public Lecture' and could not be deterred from her opinion that it was not research, *only* lectures! Who would have thought that one had to be so careful? And who would have described research lectures as *only* lectures!

But anyway, returning to the promotion problem for lawyers. Once this career information about top lawyers at the time of their tenure was placed before the committee, it could instantly see the differences in careers between, say, legal academics and economics academics. The economists could now understand the nature of the academic legal market place, while the lawyers could now understand the academic economics market place. The committee meetings became almost blissful!

Similar understandings were obtained for most of the other committees. Such simple changes, like making clear the differences in the different parts of the academic and professional market places, so improved the workings of the committees.

Dismissal: Poisoned Chalice Number Three

Perhaps the most interesting case in which I have been involved was something different again.

A reasonably senior individual had been appointed in mid-career from overseas. Usually such an appointment would be made directly at a tenured level. Certainly, each time that I have moved, I had tenure from day one. I never had to ask for it; they knew I would not have moved without it. Why would I? Why would anyone? (Of course, the security of tenure does not exist today!). This had never been a problem for me. If a new university wanted me, that was one of the things they had to do. But this had not been done for this individual; he was required to pass the tenure barrier within three years!

During his first two years, as his Executive Dean, I supported his annual reports. I had no reason not to. In addition to research, publications and graduate students, he had produced a well-cited book in his area and was even an invited contributor to a major academic encyclopedia (a signal honor). (Later, the high quality of his work was attested to by letters from distinguished academics throughout the world.)

My term as Dean came to an end and I returned to my academic department as I had done twice before. What happened next therefore did not involve me.

Attempts were made to deny him tenure after the end of his third year. This is never an easy task. The case rumbled on for a number of years. Eventually, however, after all allowable appeals, and at the final university level, his tenure was denied.

However, he continued to fight. He fought it first through the external ruling body of the university, then through the 'examiner' to the university — a most unusual step — and finally through a legal process.

Of course, I had only been involved early in the piece by supporting the first two of his annual reports. The later actions, denial of tenure and the various appeals had come long after I had stepped down from my administrative appointment. However, years later, the legal process wanted to go back to the very beginning, so I was required to appear before them. Their question came: "Why had I supported him with the two initial reports?" I gave my reasons.

The story gets more complicated. This individual was a homosexual (long before LGBTQ+), and his Head of Department, who was pushing for denial of tenure, was a lesbian. He had had to act as Head of Department in his first year when she was on sabbatical leave. During that period as the Acting Head, he had received curious complaints about the real Head from both students and staff. As Dean, I, too, kept receiving such complaints!

Believing all this to be somewhat beyond my abilities and responsibilities, and obtaining the agreement of my student and staff informants, I had, each time, referred these discussions to the officer for equity matters, the officer in charge of personnel and the head of the university.

However, the final legal process could find nothing in my files about my actions. As soon as I had left the Deanship, my files had been 'cleaned' by the central administration. There seemed to be no evidence! So, the legal process wanted to know: did I have *any* written evidence?

I said:

"As it happens, there is, but I am not sure that it would be considered evidence."

They said they would determine that!

I explained how, those several years before, as the various staff and students came to complain to me over a period of weeks, I was flabbergasted. When I came home each day, my wife would be agog to hear the latest parts of the story, especially whom I had seen, what I had been told and whom I had informed.

She, with her Librarian's Soul, said each time:

"No 'drinkies' until you have written it down."

So, each time I wrote down what had been reported to me, what discussions I had had and whom I had informed, all on separate sheets of yellow paper, sometimes A4 and sometimes legal, in my own horrible handwriting. A pig's breakfast of a report! But my wife made me date each sheet.

When I told the legal process what Eleanor and I had done all those years before, they became very excited.

"Do you still have those notes?"

they asked,

"The very fact that they are scrappily hand written, means that they count as contemporaneous evidence!"

Indeed, we still had them. They had been written at home, so I was asked to bring them in; those notes formed their most important evidence. I suspect they much helped their determination.

The first of the matters, the question of tenure, was determined on behalf of the complainant. It was judged that the tenure denial should be reversed.

Sadly, at this point, the complainant died. The coroner's report implied strongly that the stress of this entire, by now, almost seven-year long process was the primary factor!

As a result, the remaining points in the examination were adjourned *sine die*. The investigation was placed in abeyance and will probably never be reopened (though I think it could be).

Such a shame that he received his tenure but not the fruits; such a shame, too, that the remaining investigation was never completed.

16 The Conscience of the University!

In some of the private universities in the USA, the Dean of the graduate school is the 'academic conscience' of the university. He or she may be the person who has to sort out all the 'dirty little problems' that are found in even the best of institutions. Average academics usually know only the small numbers that occur in their own area, but the Graduate Dean usually knows them for the whole university!

As a result, he or she knows just how widespread such problems are.

Failing a Student!

Thus, as Graduate Dean, I had to sign off on failed graduate students. One department wanted to fail a student's Master's thesis. But on reading the case I realized that he had been a Master's student for *almost ten — yes, ten — years!* How could this have happened?

I naturally looked at the thesis, but could not really appreciate it because I was not familiar with the discipline. So of course, I enlisted help. It transpired that, indeed, it was not a very good thesis. It possibly should have been failed!

However, how can one fire a student after ten years? If he was to have been fired at all, it should have been after one year! And if he was not fired, then he should have at least had help!

A little more investigation revealed that this student had taught the first-year undergraduate courses, which is a pernicious habit in many US universities given that it is a task that the academics did not want! Though the department had supported him for ten years, he clearly had been 'used'. If we really had fired him after ten years, someone — probably me — should have been 'sued'.

So, I overturned the departmental decision. After all, not every Master's thesis can be superb; some, though mediocre, may be good enough. Maybe I'm wrong, but after allowing for ten years of work, surely the thesis must be passed!

Failing a Professor!

Another department voted to deny tenure to an assistant professor at the end of her second three-year term. Such cases also came to the Graduate Dean.

When I perused the case, I saw that she had published what I thought was a respectable number of publications (I seem to remember more than 10, not that the number is the only criterion), and she had also written a book! Of course, I could not judge the quality as it was not my discipline, but there was decent quantity. To me, it seemed like a pretty good record.

It turned out, however, that in addition to six years as an assistant professor with what I thought was a reasonable publishing and teaching record, she had been voted (as an untenured person!) into the departmental chair during her second assistant professor term! She was not very good at it and had, probably inadvertently, annoyed most of the tenured members. Of course, it was a very small department with only four tenured professors. None of them wanted the administration. Hence her, in my opinion, unfair appointment to the chair! What was to be done?

First, I checked the files for the records of the tenured staff of that department at the time when they became tenured. Not one of them had more than four publications at their time of tenure. *Whoa!* Of course, to be honest, judging them that way would not be really fair because all had been tenured a long time ago when the standards were probably lower!

Second, I gradually realized that she was in a different area of the discipline than the other four. It was an area denigrated by them; such hostilities are common in academia!

Finally, I realized that much of her work involved the contributions of women to the discipline. This was anathema to the four old men!

I denied their denial.

But, of course, it would have been no good tenuring her in such a small department with four senior colleagues who did not want her. Luckily there was another unit, also in the graduate school, into which she could fit. That head was very happy to have her, while she was very happy to move. So, the move was made.

Shortly afterwards, the original department came to me requesting to fill the vacant position. "Oh no," I said, "when I moved her over, I moved the money too."

They were so angry with me!

The Dean and the Punter

On one of my first decanal days during the summer vacation (I had started in July), I came in to discover an assistant with a huge pile of paper on her desk and a mournful look on her face. Being new, I asked:

"What's the problem?"

"Well, it's all these cases. I have to do them over the next few days."

"I'm new;" I said,

"I'm not doing anything yet; I'll give you a hand. What are they about?"

"Oh,"

she said,

"they are petitions from undergraduate students, petitioning to take graduate courses."

"Good, I'm all in favor of really good undergrads taking graduate courses,"

I said.

So, I took the top half-dozen petitions and started to look at them. The first was from an undergraduate petitioning to take a graduate course in cinema entitled 'History of Animation in the Cinema'. The second petition was similar. (Being so close to Hollywood, we had a very strong cinema school. Several of the top Hollywood producers, like Steven Spielberg, George Lucas and Stanley Kubrick, had been associated with us, either as prior students or as patrons.)

But there was no indication on either petition as to why the undergraduates wanted to take this graduate course, no evidence of their undergraduate record. I telephoned the cinema department to find out.

I heard the person on the other end of the phone cover the mouthpiece with her hand (but I could still hear what she said) and she whispered (in horror!) to someone else:

"It's — it's — it's — it's the new Graduate Dean. He — he — he — he wants to know about those two football students."

It turned out that the first two cases I had looked at were from two students on the football team petitioning to take a postgraduate course that, I discovered, had another title: 'From Krazy Kat to Charlie Brown'. Football students needed only to attend the cartoons for a 'Gentleman's C'!

What is more, it turned out that they were not petitioning to take it in the future; they had already taken it the previous semester and were petitioning to have it count! So, I denied the petitions.

What I did not know, not being an American at that point, was that although one student was an ordinary player who mainly sat on the bench, the other was the university punter — the best they had. Neither did I know that because he had already done the course the previous year, if I denied the petition, the legitimacy of the team's previous record might be called into question!

My decision caused ructions.

Within a couple of days, a large oversight committee, normally meeting only once a year to rubber-stamp football matters, was called into emergency action. I was summoned to appear before them and spent the best part of an hour explaining my decision. They turned it down. **So much for the great powers of the Graduate Dean!**

At least, however, the committee came to understand my concern. The best result I could get was the appointment of an academic person to oversee the academic careers of football students!

Perhaps, then, a small win!

'Stealing' from Oneself

Then there was a problem in one of the professional schools. It had special difficulties.

There were a very large number of graduate students. One staff member actually had over a hundred! How does one person supervise a hundred graduate students? He gave courses with imposing-sounding titles. But when 'translated', they were: 'How to Write the Introduction to Your Thesis', 'How to Write the Materials and Methods …', 'How to Write the Discussion …', etc, etc, etc.

There were even problems with the publications lists in the CVs of some of the staff. Some publications lists were puffed up (naughty, naughty), and some papers even contained a high proportion of self-plagiarism — the first time I had come across this interesting academic crime!

Worst of all, the school had a deal with the local industry. Someone from lower administrative levels could swap over into the school as assistant professor, someone from mid-levels as associate professor, someone from senior levels as full professor, and the swaps could be made in reverse. This was known within the senior levels of the school administration, not generally within the university.

Clearly this had to be sorted out, and it seems that it had been left until a new Graduate Dean (me) came in. The first part of the solution was to get to know the academic staff. The second part was to appoint a committee, what else. The most important third part was to find a chair of committee who could handle such a difficult problem with sympathy but rigor. There was such a person in the university. I was most lucky that she was willing to act.

After a little while, it was all settled.

Of course, a dean had to go, and another had to be appointed from outside the discipline. But this was all achieved.

Real Stealing!

A close colleague burst into the Graduate Dean's office with my assistant on his coattails almost trying to hold him back. He looked very angry and he threw two books across my desk.
"What are you going to do about those?"
he roared. He was already in a fury.

I slowly calmed him down. It turned out that he had been asked to do a prepublication review of a book by a press. But the book was very similar to a book written by a close colleague.
"Let me read them and I will get back to you,"
I said.

Two days later I was able to report to him that yes, the preprint was about 80% similar to the already published book. The main difference was that the pictures were in color — a new possibility at that time — and probably not available to the original author.

What to do? Happily, I did nothing because within days, I discovered that the press had withdrawn the book. They must have smelt a rat! Why did I not keep the two books? Together they might be worth money!

The Most Important Story for the Conscience of the University!

The most important first step that I had to make when I became Graduate Dean was to appoint an Associate Graduate Dean. Obviously, this is a very important appointment, not only for the Dean, but also for the graduate school and, indeed, the entire university. We had a list of good applicants and a good search committee. But the decision was mine (in those days, but not today, I'd imagine!).

It was quite a difficult matter. I am a scientist, and the science departments expected that I would appoint another scientist — and we had some good candidates. Furthermore, this was especially important at that point because the university was aiming to boost its science, technology and engineering areas. But I felt that it might be rather important for the Associate Dean to come from another quite different area of the university from me.

It happened that there was a very good candidate (in my opinion) who was from the general area of the humanities. Indeed, his doctoral thesis was on the literature of some Caribbean Islands, even involving voodoo and related matters! This was totally new to me, but I was intrigued; I decided he would be the best appointment.

At this point I realized that there were mutterings in the dovecotes. Why had Oxnard, a scientist and medic, appointed someone from the humanities? But that was not all.

Why had Oxnard appointed a woman (because though I used the words 'his thesis' and 'his appointment', that was merely a literary trick in my text)? And there was more.

Why had Oxnard appointed a black woman? And why, as it transpired, one from 'the wrong side of the tracks in the deep south'?

Of course, I am talking about Ruth Simmons. She accepted our offer, and she proved to be superb.

Three years later, Ruth and I discussed her further career possibilities. I suggested that, after her experience as Associate Dean with us, she should move to a major appointment in the East. I even predicted to her that she would eventually become President of a very good liberal arts college.

Everyone knows what happened next. Indeed, she went to Princeton in a Vice-Presidential position, then on to President of Smith College (a very good liberal arts college).

Here is where my forecasting fell short — I did not foresee that she would further move on to being President of Brown (a major university).

Ruth and I have remained in sporadic contact over the years. She invited Eleanor and I to her inauguration as President of Smith (and we had known a prior President of Smith, who was an Australian). Later she invited us to her inauguration at Brown. Finally, we were invited to her retirement celebrations from Brown. In all of those invitations, it was evident to Eleanor and I just how good she had been for those institutions, for their staff and students, and for helping solve some of the big problems those institutions had!

What a wonderful outcome for me, as I have moved from 'mentee' to mentor and to retiree. And a what a wonderful story of what should be the proper relationships among staff and students in universities.

17 Military Interludes!

Chapter

The University Air Squadron

When I was a medical student, and impressed by what I knew of my father's work on the spitfire before and during the war, I decided that I would like to join the university air squadron. There were two attractions.

One was learning to fly chipmunks. They were the first training planes for the air squadron, with the expectation of progressing on to flying other planes later. The second was that the air squadron had the best bar in the university! I was, of course, influenced by a friend in 'digs' with me; he was already in the air squadron.

I can well remember us discussing, far into the night, such burning questions (why do questions always 'burn'?) like: how many ping pong balls would render the Bismarck unsinkable?

I applied and took the written examinations. This included a number of tests that involved interesting questions, mostly mechanical. I did extremely well, getting very high marks. All went well until I got to the final interview.

An older and much bemedalled individual said:
"You are a medical student aren't you. Medical students in the RAF become doctors. You should not be learning to fly. Case dismissed!"
I was upset, but there was nothing I could do.

However, two years later I won a scholarship that allowed me to transfer out of medicine into the final year of a science degree. Aha, I thought, I'm not a medical student now. So, I applied again for the air squadron. And again, I got through the examinations to the last interview!

My heart dropped: the same cantankerous interviewer was there.

"I see you are a science student now,"

he said, recognizing me.

"But you will be rejoining medicine next year. We don't want doctors flying. Case dismissed."

Admiral in a Great Navy!

Among other wonderful things about academia are the colleagues we meet and the travels we make over the years. At the University of Birmingham, one of my colleagues in anatomy was David Brynmor Thomas. Originally training at University College, London, he later became a University of Bristol research student. Together with Professors Metcalf and Yoffey, he was interested in blood formation. David later moved to anatomy in Birmingham where we first met, and many years later he had the Chair in St. Andrews.

Eleanor and I later visited the Thomases in St. Andrews several times. It was David who put me up for Fellowship at the Royal Society of Medicine (FRSM), and I have since become an Honorary Life Fellow. It is a useful place to stay and work when back in London. Once again, wheels within wheels.

Years after Birmingham, David's mentor, Ken Metcalf had emigrated to the USA and took the Chair of Anatomy in Omaha, Nebraska. David had continued his contacts with Ken, even to the point of doing new work on blood and marrow as a visitor in

Oak Ridge, USA, using radioactive methods. When he knew I was in the USA, David gave my name to Ken. As a result, I received an invitation to give the prestigious Latta Lecture in Omaha. Dr. Latta had been the Doyen of Anatomy in Omaha!

After the lecture, a special ceremony confirmed my appointment as: Admiral in the Great Navy of the State of Nebraska.

This appointment called me to:

"diligently assume the duties of Admiral by doing and performing all manner of things thereto belonging,

to strictly charge and require all officers, seamen, tadpoles and gold-fish under my command to be obedient to my Orders as Admiral.

I am to observe and follow from time to time such directions as I shall receive according to the Rules and Discipline of the Great Navy of the State of Nebraska.

Given under my hand in the City of Lincoln, State of Nebraska, this 27th day of August, 1987, Kay Avonne Orr, 36th Governor of Nebraska."

Kay Orr was Nebraska's first female governor. Landlocked as the state is, the ship of state, figured at the base of the diploma, is a covered wagon!

It is, of course, a spoof, but a very high-class spoof, with the Governor's signature and seal attached. That diploma hangs on my wall to this day.

Ken's son sent us a photograph of David and Ken taken late in life, at a restaurant in Ponsart in the Brecon Beacons in Wales in 2017. Unfortunately, on enlargement, the picture is too pixelated. But the quart of beer in the middle is clear!

Eleanor and I knew David's Wales, especially North Wales, well. We had many holidays there. Eleanor's mother was

Welsh-speaking, and yet I speak more Welsh than El does. It was a matter of honor; I can still recite, for instance, Arglwydd Yw Yy Mugail, ni fydd eisiau arnaf. (The Lord's my shepherd, I'll not want). However, El can properly pronounce the full name of Llanfair PG: Llanfairpwllgwyngyllgogerychwyrndrobwllllantysiliogogogoch!

We went to Beddgelert (Gelert's Grave) for our honeymoon in February, 1969. We were on the top of Snowdon five times in a fortnight. The sun was bright and the air clear, even though the snow was deep and the little lake's frozen over (it *was* February after all). Of course, we didn't climb; we walked.

So, the world changes. But my memories, unlike my eyes, still seem to be sharp. I have an intention tremor of my right hand; it does not stop me from writing, though the cursor on the screen wobbles. Thank goodness, I am in anatomy and not surgery; my patients don't complain!

Brigadier General for a Day!

Many things in administration are fun. At the University of Southern California, we had lots of programs on military bases. Of course, those students can't easily travel to the university to get their degrees, and the President of the university can't travel to all the bases to confer them! Hence the senior administrators took a share of conferring degrees on the bases.

Came the day when it was my turn. I had to go to Hickam Air Force Base, Hawaii, and Kadena Air Force Base, Okinawa.

The two degree ceremonies were delightful. The number of servicemen getting degrees was very small, so the ceremonies were very personal — it wasn't just a handshake and congratulations. I was able to chat with each student. Of course, most of the students were married — so both graduand and spouse went up to receive the diploma.

Given those days, the graduands were all men, the spouses were women, and there were several babies. So, we gave three diplomas to some groups: a PhD (Doctor of Philosophy) to a graduand, a PhT (Putting Hubby Through) to a wife and, when a small child was carried up in arms, a miniature diploma, a PuP (Putting Up with Parents) for the kid! Afterwards we had celebratory parties, all very informal yet very civilized!

There was a special moment at one of the bases. We were lined up to process in. The procession consisted of the Chaplain who led the procession, me as the Acting President and degree conferrer, an Associate Provost (who was 'minding' me on behalf of the university), the Base Officer, and a few teachers who were located on the base. As we processed, up started the music: Elgar's *Pomp and Circumstance*. But of course, we were a short procession, so we were done on the podium after just a few bars.

But the music continued on... and on... and on.

Then I noticed the Chaplain waving surreptitiously at someone in the back of the hall who was obviously in charge of the canned music but who had forgotten to turn it off. Eventually he realized the problem.

The Chaplain made a short announcement, and then said we would now have the national anthem. At first nothing happened; more arm waving. Then the guy at the back got the message and pressed the button.

Up came further portions of *Pomp and Circumstance*. Yet more arm waving. Eventually he got it on to the *Star-Spangled Banner*. A very happy and informal ceremony, full of smiles, followed.

But I was next to the Chaplain. I could hear him swearing long and hard over — not under — his breath. I never knew Chaplains had such flowery vocabularies!

The end of this episode was when I got back to the university. A colleague, who had himself been in the US Armed Services, asked me what rank I was. I said:

"I have no idea; how would I know?

He said:

"Go and look at your sailing papers; that will tell you."

I said:

"I didn't sail, I flew."

"Never mind,"

he chuckled,

"your sailing papers are the memo that told you which plane to catch to get there. Come back and tell me what the GS number on the memo was."

So, I did.

"GS 17,"

I said.

He almost salaamed in front of me. That means you were a Brigadier General.

"No,"

I said,

"it can't be that, they were air force visits."

"Ah,"

he said,

"as a civilian going on base, you would have been given what is called a 'civilian-equivalent rank', and that is always an army rank!"

Why was I ranked so highly? It is partly a comparative matter, related to what your salary is in civilian life, and as the Dean of the graduate school and a medic in a top private university, my salary was very high, whereas salaries in the armed services at that time were very low.

However, it was also related to a bit of service protocol. In addition to conferring the degrees, I was, theoretically, also assessing our programs on the base. In order to do that, I had to have access to the files, and in order to have access, I had to outrank the ranking officer on the base! No wonder I was not allowed even to open a door by myself; each time I had to go through a door, a young chap with gold braids would jump out and open the door for me. So often did something like this occur that I began to think that if I even went to the loo, he would jump out and want to hold it for me!

My Draft Card

This was not my first contact with the military in the US. Of course, in the UK, I had never been in the army. I should have been drafted at 18, but was deferred because I was a medical student. When I qualified as a doctor, I became eligible for the draft again as the military was short of doctors. Yet I was again deferred (now age 24) because I was doing research for a PhD. At the end of the doctorate, at 27, yet again I should have been drafted as a physician. But that was the year they stopped the draft!

When we emigrated to the USA, of course I was not a US Citizen, but because I had been appointed to a tenured position, I was, from day one, a resident alien (with little green pointy ears!). Was I liable for the military draft? I thought I was safe. I knew the draft in the USA ceased at age 26. What I did not know, however, was that this was so for everyone except doctors. Doctors were eligible up to the birthday of their 36th year! The US military needed doctors. We are all familiar with — and enjoyed — MASH. So, I had to register for the draft, which I did.

But I was never called. Why? Certainly, the military would prefer to send a resident alien to the frontlines than a citizen.

I suspect it was because I was strictly correct when I registered. Where it asked for my degrees, I put down my English medical degrees: MB, ChB (not MD, the American medical degree!). Not reading Latin, I am sure the military thought those degrees meant something like Master of Biology and Bachelor of Chiropody.

I still have my draft card. I never did burn it as did so many other young men in those days.

Part 5

Challenging Beyond the Drawbridge

Chapters 18–22

My original mentor, Solly Zuckerman, was a science practitioner who challenged science. But he was also a science advisor who challenged governments. This had major effects on my career and those of many others of his students!

Though originally appointed Professor of Anatomy in Birmingham before the war, Solly Zuckerman's appointment as Scientific Advisor to Combined Operations during the war meant that he did not take up the Professorship until war's end. After the war, while still professor, he became Chief Science Advisor to the Government, and even in retirement, was Science Advisor in the House of Lords. We were all touched by this aspect of his life. The effect on me continued even though, over the years, I moved from the UK to the USA and then to Australia.

Because my moves crossed national borders, I could never have made the really wide contributions that might have been possible if I had stayed in one country. I could only always be 'on the edges', being primarily involved in a research, teaching and practice career. I obviously was interested, as he was, in 'challenging within the ivory tower' and changing how universities work. But I was never directly involved, as he was, 'outside the drawbridge'.

Now, in retirement, I am looking more and more outside the walls. I am seeing more clearly the longstanding damages, both internal and external, that have been visited upon research and learning, upon students and teachers, upon schools and universities, upon science and medicine (and many other disciplines), by administrations and governments. Though these damages are longstanding, they are now enormously magnified by the coronavirus pandemic.

Yet in retirement (1997), I also found myself at the beginning of what has transpired to be a further quarter of a century of personal researches with continuing research funding, increased collaborations with international colleagues, ever more scientific publishing, some continued teaching, and all with no administration! If you still can, why wouldn't you?

Accordingly, at retirement, I never took up the 'And Now Beyond the Drawbridge' idea. Perhaps that was a mistake! Perhaps, though it is now too late for me, it is not too late for my younger colleagues, my students, their parents, our wider society, and this book!

Chapter 18: Science Advice: From Axes and Arrows to Pandemics and 'Cyber-Demics'

Chapter 19: Do We have a Science/Technology/Medicine Problem?

Chapter 20: Halfway through the Drawbridge: Climbing Up, Sliding Down!

Chapter 21: Are Teaching and Research Careers Now Moribund?

Chapter 22: The World Sphere: Should We Be Worried?

18 Science Advice: From Axes and Arrows to Pandemics and 'Cyber-Demics'

Chapter

Part of the excitement of being at medical school with Solly Zuckerman was related to his links outside the university. Of course, it was all very secret!

The idea that science and medicine can have vital influences in peace and war has a long and venerable history. The middens of prehistoric flint-knapping sites tell us not only about the earliest tools, but also about the earliest weapons (axeheads and arrowheads). Archimedes (the ancient mathematician and astronomer) designed defensive fortifications and attacking engines. Leonardo da Vinci and Michelangelo (so well-known to us as artists) were also 'merchants of death', inventing 'instruments of defence and attack'. The earlier weapons and tactics of war seem always to have taken full advantage of whatever the combination of the sciences, crafts, and arts could produce, the fruits of the so-called less divided cultures.

Then, later, a divorce occurred between scientist and soldier, between scientific and military affairs. Where it was the habit of the soldier to obey without question, it was that of the scientist to question without obeying! A gulf arose.

This new gulf started to close in the early 20th century. The First World War was a particular turning point. It saw the emergence of submarine warfare (though there were some wooden submarines in the previous century), aerial offensives (though there had been earlier attempts at balloon reconnaissance), and tanks (possibly descendants of the testudo of ancient Greek and Roman times [testudo: a turtle]; indeed, the first tanks were something like turtles). These transitions were powerfully influenced by men like Tizard and Lindemann, and scores of others who became engaged in the technical backing of the armed services.

Amongst the earliest of these 'men', even before the First World War and initially forced upon reluctant government departments and a reluctant military, was Florence Nightingale and her statistical (pie chart) descriptions of how thousands lived, fought and died in the Crimea! She received from Queen Victoria the first Order of Merit, for which the criterion was that it could only be held at any one time by 24 living English**men**!

This involvement of non-military advisors in the military efforts of the UK dwindled after the war to end all wars! It was variously rekindled as the signs of another European clash became ever more thinkable. Instead of being just a standby to provide for military needs as demanded by the soldier, the scientist began to suggest what these needs might be. The idea of a 'death ray' (after the Flash Gordon of my childhood Saturday mornings) seems reminiscent of the detection and location of aircraft by radio methods (radar). The ideas of *Mr. Tompkins in Wonderland* and *Mr. Tompkins Explores the Atom*, both my favorite boyhood readings, were descriptive of the coming enormous power of the atomic bomb.

This all represented a change in the relationship between scientific ideas and military control. It led to 'operational research'. This was not really a new idea, but putting it into such powerful practice certainly was!

The result of all this, largely channelled by war, was the development of a cadre of 'advisors' (even humanists and artists, as well as mathematicians, scientists and engineers) who had ideas for military advances, and who gradually learnt (to a degree) how to work with the military. This was 'new learning' for these 'new individuals'. The war lasted long enough that a 'new expertise' in science and technology advising gradually developed. This led to the additional career that Zuckerman, among many others, took up.

Science Advising in War

Zuckerman's expected pre-war move from Oxford to become Professor of Anatomy in Birmingham was thus postponed until after the war. He eventually entered the war effort, becoming Military Advisor to Winston Churchill and Dwight Eisenhower.

He early on explored the wounding effects of explosions, which became crucial as the air raids on Britain stepped up. Thus, he conducted experiments determining how many two-dimensional plastic 'rabbits' placed at different distances from controlled explosions were toppled. This was simple stuff! (We had those 'rabbits' still scattered around the Birmingham department).

He carried out similar experiments with plastic 'men', simulating soldiers in the standing, kneeling and lying positions of the 'lead' soldiers of my childhood. (Naturally these were called 'zuckermen'.)

He studied casualties from city bombings and exploded military myths as to why people died. It was not from blast compressing the exterior of the chest, nor from blast passing down the trachea and exploding the chest internally (favorite contrary hypotheses of the military!). Instead, they died because the walls fell on them (shades of Jericho!). A side effect of this was the design of a civilian defence helmet (naturally known as the Zuckerman Helmet).

He quickly realized that bombing did not render the civilian population fearful. Quite the reverse: after a raid, those who could would pick themselves up, raise their fists to the bombers in the sky, and go back to war work with redoubled efforts!

Later, in Northern Africa/Southern Europe, he was responsible for the planning and analysis of air operations. One effort was like a scientific experiment, exploring how to invade Sicily using the small island of Pantelleria (Operation Corkscrew) as the 'laboratory animal'. This resulted in the development of policies aiding the breakdown of enemy communications in Sicily and Southern Italy (policies privately known by his opponents as 'Zuckerman's Folly' when later used in the lead-up to the Normandy Landings). (I wrote my thesis on a sit-up and beg typewriter that had been with one of Zuckerman's assistants, Barney Campion, throughout North Africa and Italy!)

The bombing business resulted in later bitter and prolonged disputes over bombing targets, even continuing long after the war.

This, then, was part of the long apprenticeship in war-time scientific advising served by Zuckerman and many of his colleagues.

Science Advising in Peace

After Zuckerman's move to Birmingham anatomy at war's end, his continued provision of defence advice to government led eventually to his appointment as Chief Scientific Advisor to the Ministry of Defence (1960 to 1964) and later Chief Scientific Advisor to the Prime Minister (from 1964 to 1971).

And even this was not the end. After retirement, he continued to advise very widely in science, technology and defence to successive Prime Ministers *of both political persuasions!* During all those years (and subsequently from the House of Lords, as Baron Zuckerman of Burnham Thorpe in the County of Norfolk) until his death in 1988, he was involved in almost every scientific, technological, medical and defence controversy.

It was on nuclear issues above all in which Zuckerman was most passionately involved. He deeply believed that we could and must stop the nuclear madness, and soon. His short book, *Nuclear Illusion and Reality*, tells us how. He combined information, opinion, science and passion in fascinating measure. Though he would cheerfully admit to instances in which his opinions were wrong, he was always worth listening to. He enjoyed those indispensable attributes: a questioning mind, scepticism of dogma, disrespect for tradition, searching tirelessly for better possibilities, but never believing that he (or anyone else) had found truth. Indeed, that falsification, not truth, was what was critical! He was a confirmed 'Popperian'.

Yet this advising career did not interfere with his continued link with anatomy and academia.

This is evidenced by the supporters on his Coat of Arms

dexter: A Great Ape (*Gorilla gorilla*)

sinister: A Tarsier (*Tarsius spectrum*)

Motto: *Quot homines tot sententiae* (so many men, so many opinions).

Scientists often have units named after them: the **pascal**, a unit of pressure named after Blaise Pascal; the **newton**, a measure of force after Sir Isaac Newton; the **farad**, a unit of capacitance after Faraday, and so on. Solly Zuckerman's name gave rise to a unit of work (a little tongue in cheek), the **milli-zuckerman**: the work done by **one man in one day!**

I myself, as consecutively medical student, research student, young physician, university research fellow, then lecturer and senior lecturer, did not directly figure in any of this advisory work. I was just a beginning anatomist. But I saw it!

I knew Zuckerman well. He was supervisor of my first undergraduate research. It frightened me to death when he came to examine my first anatomical dissections with a large magnifying glass! And my direct colleague, Dr. Eric Ashton, was also involved in what was then government-classified work on the abilities of dogs to detect mines. So, of course, I knew a little of what was going on outside.

We were all, naturally, proud of our relationship with someone so high in government circles. Notwithstanding this, Solly never took up government work full time; he always insisted, even in his retirement years, even after his elevation to the House of Lords, in remaining a professor and continuing basic research with academic colleagues (of whom I was one).

Thus, I visited the UK almost every year after my move to the USA. Usually I would meet with him at Regents Park (his London Zoological Society office). Once or twice I had to meet him in his defence office in Whitehall. What a picnic that was, going through security there. I continued to work with him, writing scientific papers with him, speaking at scientific meetings he organized, and I was even involved in a textbook with him. Indeed, he proposed our next collaboration just some few weeks before his death.

In all of this he was always supported by his medical school and university. Such support was often provided in those days to their staff. I, myself, have been a recipient many times.

Science Advice AZ to the UK Government (AZ = After Zuckerman)

After Zuckerman, what then happened to scientific and medical advice to government? Zuckerman's services in advising the government was continuous over four decades! Many of his scientific peers gave similar continuous support. They handled such support while remaining academics!

In contrast, after Solly's death, this continuity was followed by:

First, two science advisors who served for only 2–3 years and to only a single Prime Minister (being replaced when each Prime Minister fell);

Next, three science advisors who had links with Prime Ministers, but only through serving as cabinet undersecretaries; and

Finally, four science advisors who had no direct links to Prime Ministers or the cabinet at all!

This was a long-continued reduction in science advice to the UK Government.

This reduction still goes on (though the frights of the coronavirus may now be tempering it)!

Most science advisors today, while certainly all excellent individuals, have not had the lifelong apprenticeship of Zuckerman and his many colleagues in those earlier times.

Science Advice in the USA: What Little I Knew!

When I moved to the USA in 1966 as a permanent resident (a green card holder), I could not expect to have any direct links to USA governmental matters.

However, I was soon involved, almost accidentally, in the design of plastic armor for the protection of helicopter personnel. Such work was obviously within the realm of anatomy: the form and proportions of the human body! But my inclusion here was to help my then Head of Department, Professor Ronald Singer (at The University of Chicago), in classified work on which **he** was engaged (I merely helped with measurements and simple statistics).

Yet the more general problems in which I became interested meant that I also learnt new methods far from those of anatomy, and many from classified work! These methods were developed by others to examine aerial pictures of jungles from the air (initially in Panama, not Viet Nam), study patterns in sections of oil-bearing rocks (at the Kansas State Geological Survey), and improve some of the earliest of the satellite photographs of the moon (NASA).

Of course, I (and everyone else) was aware of the importance of the war-time and early post-war science advice in the USA. We all knew of Vannevar Bush's involvements in the Manhattan Project, Philip Handler's work in setting up the National Science Foundation, and George Marshall's invention of the Marshall Plan. These were three individuals (along with many others) who were high up in advising USA governmental policies, and highly successfully. This was continued by scientists who were involved in nuclear radiation and the bomb.

But my own direct knowledge of science advising in the USA relates to a later period when I was Graduate Dean at the University of Southern California. I came to know Jack Marburger, the physicist and Undergraduate Dean there. After a stellar career in physics, Jack became involved in various activities in science advising to the government. Eventually he was appointed as Science Advisor to the first President Bush. What then happened?

Initially, Marburger was located in the White House with an office next to President Bush and the ability to walk in to see Bush at any time.

Then he was removed to a corner office, away from the President.

After this, he was demoted to a separate building far down Pennsylvania Avenue.

Later still, he was required to report to the President only through the White House media!

Finally, the White House media apparatus would change (without reference back to him) crucial elements of his reports!

And during President Trump's time, advice on science and medicine was removed from the White House horizon. Trump required his White House media apparatus to eliminate phrases such as *evidence-based, climate effects, eggs and embryos, fetal development, human reproduction, immunization and vaccination*, etc.

The almost total reduction of science advice to government in the USA mirrors the same trend that had occurred previously in the UK after Zuckerman:!

Science Advice in Australia: I Know Nothing!

Of course, though now an Australian citizen, I am very much a 'Johnny come lately'. I have no long-term Australian academic experience behind me, so I could not be involved directly. But I am an observer of the scene, and the following is what I see:

The first Chief Scientist in Australia advised the **Prime Minister**.

The second Chief Scientist advised only the **cabinet**.

The next four Chief Scientists were only **part-time** (one of them only one day per week!).

One recent Chief Scientist said, rather optimistically, of science and medicine research as:

"We do not have a train wreck."

But he also said that Australia was:

**"The only OECD country without a science
or technology strategy."**

One also recently resigned after only two years, citing the **ineffectiveness of *her* position!**

More recently still, science advising in Australia was moved **from a major ministry to a minor ministry**.

Most recently of all, it has been located **completely outside the cabinet**!

Do not misunderstand me. There have been, and still are, some truly excellent individuals involved in advising in science, technology and medicine in Australia. They have provided very good reports on various problems (health, disability, ageing, poverty, inequity, climate, energy, pollution, and especially recently, fires, droughts, storms, floods and the coronavirus pandemic). But most of such reports remain on the shelves and result in no action, save for more requests for further reports from other advisors on the same problems, which are then likewise shelved!

So how has this happened? First, the science advisors of today have not had the long apprenticeship in science advising that war time produced in earlier British and US scientists!

Second, a larger part of the problem is that present-day governments do not understand the dangers of choosing only the advice that supports their own ideological persuasions. *The earlier British and American advisors served governments of all colors: a critical element of independence!*

Third, science and medicine has been greatly depleted of governmental support almost everywhere in the West and particularly in Australia, and this is especially evident in comparisons with some societies in the East.

Is it possible that the beginning coronavirus problems, which highlight the need to find urgent national answers and a complementary need to avoid the worldwide economic difficulties of those answers, are the latest and worst effects of the demotion of science advice to governments?

Yet there is some sign that the more recent fear of pandemics (attack of the viruses) is changing things. But I also worry that this may turn out to be temporary, that as soon as the immediate fears are over, it will be back to taking little notice of scientific, technical and medical advice — back to the era of political polarization and ideological fixation!

Furthermore, there is also the fear of 'cyber-demics' (attack of the computers). We are not defending ourselves appropriately against them (see another chapter). As a result, governments are becoming afraid, very afraid.

As a further immediate result of the pandemic, advisors are being heard a little bit more! Yet even this hearing improvement is not what it seems. In this arena, as in most others, governments pick and choose, but only on the basis of what suits their immediate philosophy, of their immediate electoral needs, and of their concerns about the next election!

It is true that governments are elected to lead and not hide behind the boffins. They must therefore weigh up the advices they are given, and they must make the decisions. But if making decisions is based on picking and choosing what suits their immediate partisan needs and wants, then we might as well have no advices at all, and we would have lost democracy!

19 Do We Have A Science/Technology/Medicine Problem?

In spite of vaccination, children throughout the world continue to die from measles. The World Health Organization blames the resurgence on low vaccination rates. Low rates are partly due to people opposing the advice to vaccinate!

Likewise, global warming (threatening the habitability of parts of the planet in the shorter term, and of the whole planet in the longer term) is worsened by scepticism about climate advice.

Further, belated government attempts to dampen the *pandemic coronavirus crashes* may be leading to a second, possibly much worse danger, *pandemic economic crashes!*

There have also been attacks by hacks (in the modern meaning of the word) on industry, on universities, on science, medicine and defence, on politics, on government, and through espionage (hackers hacking the hackers!). Is this a third pandemic, a *'cyberdemic'?* China's 'digital attack economy' amounted, in 2017, to about 30% of its gross domestic product. In contrast, Australia's 'cyber army' may possibly be 76,000 recruits by 2024!

So, aren't rising sea levels, increasing heat waves, fires and droughts, use of fossil fuels, pollutions of land, river, sea, air and space, interferences with many aspects of medicine (especially arguments against vaccinations for childhood diseases and other epidemics) and the loss of plant and animal life due to human interference with the environment — which is the ultimate interrogation of the Earth's web of life — the reality that we should know?

And what about some even more recent matters on which science advice to governments may be important? One weakness for Australia is our vulnerability to economic attacks. Why are we not quietly widening our range of customers? Are we leaving ourselves vulnerable by being too dependent upon one customer?

These weaknesses have become more and more serious in recent times. Cyber attacks upon businesses come not only from criminals after money, but from business competitors after ideas and from national governments after power.

Of course, it is not easy for Australia (or the USA, Europe or much of the rest of Asia) to tackle these problems. Alone among the nations of the world, China's national and overseas companies, China's science and scientists, China's military (both open and hidden), and even many Chinese overseas emigrants who are beholden to the Chinese Communist Party are persuaded, directed, or even compelled to hand data to the government, including data held in the cloud!

In particular, China is betting on artificial intelligence (AI). It is investing and deploying AI on a scale not replicated by any other country; not even the USA, and certainly not Australia. All of this has profound geopolitical implications!

As AI technologies drive debates over values like surveillance and privacy, free speech and censorship, conflicts seem to be inevitable. Science advisors in Washington working with both the US and UK governments have noted:

> *"This is a challenge. Whoever implements them first*
> *and best will gain advantage."*

And, perhaps, there are other issues to do with the specifics of these new digital technologies that we do not know. It may take AI to know how the AI race will go!

China is **strongly** accelerating its investments in AI (and related science, technology and engineering). The West (in its various countries) is not!

China's acceleration (an acceleration denied in the West) is because of the powers of its central government to take advice, marshal data, mandate actions and employ resources. China's government is providing billions in funding for startups, launching major programs to woo researchers to return from overseas, secretly streamlining its data policies and modifying the work of overseas colleagues, both those who are ethnically Chinese and those who are not! China has produced, for example, internal population controls (such as AI news-reading and face identification), AI-powered strategies for external relations and AI applications (perhaps most alarming) for military and espionage purposes! Western universities are one port of entry.

The USA has started to understand this problem, tackling it by overseeing Chinese investments, banning technological business with Chinese firms, becoming wary of Chinese equipment and aiming to prosecute data and technology theft.

But these now are less useful answers than they might have been earlier. Though borrowing and stealing still go on, China now has no real need to depend on them. China has been following pathways like those of prior countries as they developed.

For example, Japan once produced poor quality gadgets by copying from the West. But that was long ago. For many years now, Japan has produced some of the best gadgets in the world.

Similarly, when I first visited China just after the end of the cultural revolution, there were almost no cars but very large numbers of bicycles. There were only two kinds of bicycles: one was a copy of the British Raleigh, the other of the British Hercules. One could tell because the Chinese had even copied the insignia at the top of the front forks in each!

But, not now! By pouring financial and brain resources into its own organizations to levels much greater than in the West, China is now producing some of the best of everything in the world, moving strongly ahead in its own right.

These developments come amid increasing political tensions. One worries about the effect of the West's responses. Are we simply accelerating China's own efforts to develop its own alternatives, further developing its own interferences in overseas industries, governments and even electorates? This race between China and the USA, which the USA is already losing, has also moved separately to other countries. They, too, are being pushed to take sides in the competition for turf.

Yet the West's faults are not just due to government. Academia is also sometimes ill-equipped to handle these problems. I have never forgotten having to support a candidate for a high tenured position in a university. He was a distinguished cryptologist, but he had gone straight into cryptology from a baccalaureate degree, so he had *'no PhD'*. The distinguished work he had done in cryptology was largely classified, so he had *'no publications'*. He therefore also had *'no academic colleagues'* who were allowed to vouch for him. **No doctorate, no publications, no references!** As he didn't fit the standards, the academic search committee wanted to turn him down.

To return to the main thesis, however, all this, given the recent strength of Chinese computers, computing power and artificial intelligence, as well as their effects on business, military and national affairs, are extremely serious. Our governments do not seem to be able to handle such problems, and our science has now been so denuded that it can scarcely help.

But what is much worse is that our science advice fails because governments act slowly, or not at all. And when they do act, it is evident that they are often acting with a particular future in mind — a future of their own desire.

I do not mean to imply that the advisors have all the answers. But I do mean to imply that advisors need a genuine seat at the table.

Our governments have to embrace the evidence-based (one of the phrases 'deleted' by Trump) realities of science. What some non-scientists (and even some scientists) believe about non-evidence-based science can be a matter of life and death.

One problem is about what constitutes scientific evidence. This is not always clear. As my earlier chapters indicate, 'real' science is often a much messier, more complicated and less straightforward process than the traditional stereotype of discovery in a dramatic 'eureka' moment. Evidence is usually accumulated gradually, and its significance is typically only 'probable', even sometimes only 'possible', but almost never 'totally certain'. The physical, chemical, biological, medical, environmental and societal processes that matter so much are themselves so messy and complicated that it is difficult to trace them in full detail.

There are many and genuine complexities in such understanding. First, scientists have access to the reality under study only through the lens of evidence-testing. Second, in many of these problems, the scientist is often part of the system being observed (as when humans study humanity). Third, what counts as scientific information is sometimes uncertain; scientific incompetence, even scientific fraud, may interfere. Fourth, the complexity is great enough that the degree to which one level of a theory is sufficiently established to be used in assessing a next level of theory may be unclear.

One common way to approach such complex natural and societal processes is by building 'models', which are sets of simplified assumptions (often in the form of mathematical equations: an immediately frightening concept to government!). While models can capture a fairly high degree of reality, they only approximate to reality out there in the 'real world' and, thus, can also be wrong under certain circumstances. Still, they give a chance of predicting where natural processes (that could make or break our futures) are going. They may help inform expectations and policy making.

These subtleties do not render scientific information either useful or useless. However, they can be mistakenly misinterpreted, or even deliberately described, as if they were mistaken.

In other words, not only must the science advising be honest, but so too must the reporting and usage of science advice! Mal-reporting and mal-usage particularly come from media misuse and government desire.

Finally, for science, technology or medicine to tell us anything, it must be heard at the top levels of government. It must be properly reported and be freed from the chains of predetermined ideas, especially from right and/or left ideologies. It must not be the creature of one side of politics. It must be relieved of the fear that universities are a breeding ground for left-wing radicals who might undermine right-wing governments, or *vice versa*. It must not suffer from the manipulation of information, the distortion of questions and the hiding of ideas.

Governments, thus, are part of the problem. The Australian government is actively antagonistic toward universities, even noticeably more antagonistic than in most other OECD countries. China in contrast is incredibly supportive of universities, pouring funding into them as though there was no tomorrow! Yet even China may now be entering a mode of negativity toward universities, education, research and research-related industries (e.g., China's very own home-grown giants, like Tencent and Alibaba, that are now being denuded of support!).

Chapter 20

Halfway through the Drawbridge: Climbing Up, Sliding Down

It was once the case that young academics (lecturers in the UK, assistant professors in the USA) would aspire to be distinguished professors. They would hope to find new knowledge and want to improve their disciplines. Most of all, they would wish for new and better students to carry on the flame. These were some of the career goals.

Today, all that has changed.

Professors today are rarely able to do these things. They are overly burdened with lower-level administration while carrying out the dictates of higher-level superiors. They can no longer develop their disciplines through appointments and promotions. Their tasks now are to dis-appoint and 'depromote'. They do not have the time, or the brief, or the support, to have any effect upon disciplinary development (one of their major functions in my day). About all that they can now do is appoint temporary part-timers!

These changes have come about as powers have moved from academics to administrators, and from the mores of collegiality to the customs of business!

As a result, universities are once again suffering a brain drain, but one different from the brain drain of my youth. In my youth, the brain drain was a pull from overseas, for example the pull by the funds available in the USA from the fund reductions in the UK.

Today, the brain drain is a push by government from research and teaching to almost anything and anywhere else! Eight of my recent students, all good students, have been so pushed away. Some of them were among the best I have ever had.

One obtained two PhDs, a first in theoretical plasma physics and a second, with me, in mathematical biology. But he was forced to become, for a number of years, a mainstay of computing in the banking world! Subsequent to that, he managed to return to his love of teaching, but as a high-level teacher in a high school. Initially good for the bank, later very good for the high school, but a major loss for the enterprise of finding new knowledge!

Another post-PhD researcher, because the university would not tenure her (she wasn't even asking for more money, just security as an academic *and* mother), took a major research position with millions of research dollars in a top laboratory in the USA (a laboratory, Novartis, whose London home I had known in earlier days).

A third, absolutely fascinated by the research she was doing, just could not secure a university position and could only land herself a series of part-time temporary posts. She stuck it out for several years — hoping — but eventually decided to take a teaching diploma and now has a high-level position in a high school, helping to encourage and prepare students with ability but needing aspiration to think of further and higher education. A 'partial win' for her, a 'major win' for that high school and its students, even a 'win' in the long term for education. But would the result have been better if she had been able to continue in university research and teaching? Possibly yes, and also possibly no; we will never know. But we do know that an excellent person was denied the career she wanted and for which she was properly prepared. And there was great angst in making the change!

Increasingly, there are now many more women appointed in academia, and this is appropriate. But increasingly, these new appointments are part time, temporary or short term. This is not good for women. And younger men are just not coming in at all. The older men in secure positions have almost all already gone!

Security in university academic appointments can only be achieved today by leaving insecure research and teaching appointments and moving to administration. Thus, first jobs in administration can lead to ongoing appointments and promotional possibilities (e.g., to graduate dean, to research provost, to deputy vice chancellor, and for a few, the top prize, principal, president or vice chancellor). Most are then lost from research and teaching!

Times have changed from the days when professors, as a group, influenced the academic direction of the university by advising vice chancellors. Academic boards now have few useful effects upon university directions. And thank goodness that is so, say many current administrators, for whom academic boards and their professors are a nuisance. We are now in a time when central administrators manage the top professors, and governments manage the top administrators, both based on holding the purse.

Times have changed from when a vice chancellor's salary was perhaps one third more than a professor's. Today's vice chancellor may receive five times a professor's salary.

These changes may be good, but I remain unconvinced. And I am looking to the next generations of students to understand these problems, and to have the creativity to fix them.

Research, Teaching and Service!

My own experiences were so different. I was greatly influenced by Solly Zuckerman (Birmingham), George Beadle and then Edward

Levi (both University of Chicago), Zohrab Kaprielian (USC, Los Angeles) and, to a lesser degree (because the contact was so short), Robert Smith (UWA, Western Australia, but an Australian who had previously been University President at British Columbia, a Canadian institution but Norte Americano in customs). These people attained top administrative positions, but they also were top academics. All maintained their direct links with the careers of staff, the development of disciplines, the futures of students *and their own academic work and ideas.*

The first of these, Solly Zuckerman, despite having a variety of positions advising prime ministers and governments on defence and science over many years, *never gave up his position as Professor.* He continued to work in his discipline for the whole of his life, including long after retirement and up to his death.

George Beadle, though Chicago President, was a Nobel winner and *remained an academic* for his entire lifetime. Edward Levi, likewise, though Dean of Law, later President of the university, and later still US Attorney General, *never truly left academia.*

I never had the possibility of such senior national positions as did Zuckerman and Levi. That was immediately precluded by my moves across three continents. But I developed my own small parallels. Thus, while I was persuaded into three Decanal positions in three universities, I always accepted them as giving service to those universities. I carried out those services with the best of intentions. But I always insisted on remaining in research and teaching, pursuing student improvements, staff careers and discipline developments!

Of course, there was always a *quid pro quo* in the Mephistophelian bargain! With the service I was asked to give, I always required that my institutions would provide me with internal research support. Importantly, in addition to that provision, I always also managed to remain in the external grantsmanship stakes! The result of teaching and researching while 'servicing' keeps the faith.

This is now almost impossible. Administration is a full-time non-academic job.

Today, in retirement, I have been even luckier. I have been able to continue the research and teaching pathway seamlessly. I have gained enormous pleasure in it. Certainly my curriculum vitae does not show any gaps in grants won, papers and books published, or students graduated. My last grant, in twenty years of retirement, was two years ago (I know there will be no more). My last research student (but is he my final?) graduated last year! My last publication (so is it my final?) is this year! And this book may not be my last book, only my next book!

Paradoxically, these seemingly intermittent part-time service periods in a largely full-time research and teaching career only served to increase my enjoyment of research and teaching! Each time I moved to a new university, it seemed to produce a new burst of creativity. Each time I went from Professor to Dean *and back*, it seemed to produce other such bursts. Every time my thoughts went to a clinical problem, it generated a scientific idea. Even just walking across campus each day, from my Dean's office in the morning to my research lab in the afternoon, cleared my mind. It is as though the stimulus of change has kept the creative research/teaching juices flowing.

Can this be done today? I wonder. *Or is it not wanted today?* That may be so!

Certainly, individuals who take up administration knowing they will return to academia are more likely to support research and teaching. Those who leave teaching and research to make administration a full-time and final career are likely to support management!

What Used to Happen! An Almost Unbelievable Story!

I have never forgotten how, shortly after I arrived in Chicago in 1966, the University was starting its first official campaign to raise money. Of course, it had been raising money for more than a century before from wonderful donors including the first Rockefeller. But an official public campaign in the 1960s? That was something quite new.

The Board of Trustees (somewhat equivalent to the Senate in Australia) debated long and hard about starting such a campaign. This led to the motion that the Board would only consider a public campaign if a third of the money could be raised *before* the campaign was announced, and if — and only if — the professoriate would support the idea by giving money to that *unannounced* campaign.

The result: the approximately 1,000 academic staff, as there were at that time, contributed an average of more than $1,000 each to the faculty campaign. And this, in the early 1960s, was at a time when faculty salaries were, and now I guess, probably around $12,000 per annum on average.

That the academic staff could or, indeed, would do this says remarkable things about their loyalty to the institution.

Imagine the academic staff of one of today's Australian universities making that kind of gift. This would be, *parri passu* with changes in salaries today, something like $20,000 or more each! What would the staff union make of that?

The Rise of the Manager

Modern universities of all kinds have now changed due to the rise of the manager. This is not special; it has occurred everywhere. Not only have managers risen in universities, they have risen in industry, they have risen in government, they have risen in the public service, they have risen everywhere. Part of this is important and inevitable. As universities have increased in complexity, new organizational guidance, new financial accountability, new specialized services, new reporting activities and new equities all need new rules and new rulers.

Is there, however, a price to pay? Academic autonomy, a voice in internal university affairs, the development of disciplines, the freedoms to teach and investigate, and the privileges of practice have all decreased. The price too often seems to be loss of loyalty.

Of course, there is no place in academia for loyalty in thinking. The task for thinking is to be disloyal, to try to show what is wrong. But there is a major place for loyalty in academia: loyalty to people, disciplines and institutions.

The Death of Loyalty?

Yet loyalty, today, is often missing! The ways that people, disciplines and institutions operate actively militate against loyalty today. So many of my younger colleagues (and I am in touch with them) feel that they are not supported by their managers and institutions. *They fear the day of the pink slip.*

In my time, it was not like that. Even in the beginning and for the rest of his life, my first professor, as I have explained elsewhere, supported me in my career to an incredible extent. His loyalty to me engendered in me reverse loyalty to him.

Further, everywhere that I have been, I have felt supported by my institutions: in Birmingham, Chicago, Southern California, Western Australia. I have always believed that this loyalty was part of what education was about.

Such loyalty generated in me reverse loyalties: to colleagues and students, to institutions, and to disciplines. Even today, in so-called retirement, I spend much time trying to cheer up my colleagues who are having second thoughts about university careers! Should this worry us? Should we not attempt to combat it?

The Corporate Model of the University

The collegiate structures of the university have gradually been converted into corporate models, though it has taken decades for that to become clearly evident. This has now become especially obvious as a result of the economic effects of the Covid-19 pandemic, the increasingly separated wings of politics and the widening gulf between the USA and China. It makes me wonder if it is time for third models; not a return to earlier roots (as many academics would like), but rather to create new ones.

Part of the reason would be to stop the large-scale redundancies in universities that are occurring almost daily. Another part would be to alleviate the reduced prospects for even the best (usually the richest) institutions. Yet another part would be to correct the almost total crises awaiting other (especially the very poorest) institutions. But perhaps the very largest part, and especially important, would be a reshaping of higher education.

The problem starts with a look at the finances of the corporate structures of the universities, which are starting to mirror those of the commercial sector.

There is increasing recourse to market-based justifications for any strategic decisions (both within individual units and at a wider corporate level). Such decisions are increasingly centralized, with little (if any) input from the professoriate. They are increasingly made without transparency, in a cone of silence, and protected by confidentiality clauses. Universities have become commercial corporations; their administrations have become boards of directors; vice-chancellors are CEOs; *professors are just employees; students are just customers*.

Such models have generated increasingly intense competition between institutions, with aggressive student recruitment, increased marketing budgets, and changes in staff activities. It has brought about a casualization of the research-teaching workforce, increased autocracy of administrators, and a cohort of well-paid managers. This dark description is not just a consequence of today's coronavirus pandemic. The pandemic is merely emphasizing changes that have been coming on for twenty years and more.

Universities (even the privates of the US) are, in general, not truly private institutions.

They are not allowed (nor should they be allowed) to fail.

They are essential services to nations, continents, and a world.

What can be done?

The Costs of the Corporate Model

The real problems are more complex than we think. They stem from changes over most of the time I have been in Australia. At the time I arrived, the top Australian universities were good because they were funded by the government for undergraduate education, postgraduate learning, and postgraduate and faculty research (endowment support was quite small). Other universities were funded for what they did: undergraduate student education with less or even no research. Since then, there has been a long period of reduction of governmental support of all types.

The top-most universities have been forced to handle this by becoming reliant, and increasingly so, on overseas student revenues. The degree of this is remarkable. For example, one major Australian university drew 34% of its students from overseas, with much higher returns than from local students. And of this 34%, some 70% came from China! This policy has increasingly produced billions of dollars for Australia's most prominent universities, attempting, but failing, to replace the lost revenues from the government. Universities had started to think of themselves as one of the very largest of Australia's 'export earners'! (Of course, the coronavirus pandemic and worries about information leakages abroad are killing that.)

What After the Corporate Model?

The original collegial model of higher education was based, *albeit only to a degree*, on three internal functions: transparency, accountability and collegiality. The present corporate model has killed the old model! So these functions have been lost. Although many especially older academics would like to return to the old model, that is no longer possible. Indeed, that desire, a return to the old model, is part of the problem now! What might be the shape of the next — and third — model? The earlier functions are still important!

In third models, could transparency be achieved by mandating that all budgetary decisions, as well as all university administrative meetings, be made public (except in cases of individual privacy)?

In third models, could accountability be enhanced by limiting the self-regulatory actions (and especially of their salaries) of the senior managers?

In third models, could collegiality, currently almost completely lost, be returned by a new reorganization of internal university structures? Such reorganization could include reducing the number of administrative levels, with closer links and smaller differentiations between the 'workers' and the 'overseers'. (In parenthesis, it is even possible that a degree of this reorganization is starting now in my own institution under our new Vice Chancellor.) Could such reorganizations allow for greater participation in selections, nominations and elections to major managerial roles?

Finally, and most importantly, could third models be properly resourced to a degree similar to that of, for example, Chinese universities?

Such a focus, produced by a collective of researchers, teachers, students and scholars, and aimed at the pursuit of research, academic inquiry, external application and advanced as well as beginning pedagogy, could be the driving forces of change.

This is not a return to the older way. It is a major change to a way that never previously existed! It is possible that it may come about through responses to the pandemic.

Epidemics, Pandemics and 'Syndemics': Further Effects on Universities

The whole world is now caught up in a perfect storm of epidemics and pandemics with resulting 'syndemics'.

For example, the epidemics of chronic diseases, new infectious diseases and public health failures (especially of aged and disabled care) combined with the Covid-19 pandemic provide a combination of medical, social and economic casualties: a global burden — a 'syndemic', to coin a term. This is changing education.

Major re-qualification was rarely considered in the old days (though continuous change did occur, or should have occurred). However, even before Covid-19, the half-life of learning was shortening. One **major** qualification in young adult life, even then, would not be enough.

Now the learning that people will need is changing even more rapidly. Relearning may need to be reimagined three, four, or even more times during a life. And superimposed upon degrees of continuous change in learning will be new discontinuities in learning. New learnings will not obviously follow on from old learnings. Some jobs will continue to need improvement and continuous change. But many jobs will not, and they will go; new jobs will require discontinuity.

This 'syndemic' is also producing changes in the mechanism of learning. For many years now, the increasing numbers of students and the reducing numbers of teachers have been forcing the use of computerized ways of providing education. But while these methods have been taken up widely and are good for some teachers and students, it is becoming evident that they are not actually very good for most. They solve the problem of having fewer teachers and more students, but they also engender boredom, place emphases on rote learning, increase ways of cheating, and discriminate against those who cannot afford the equipment.

Much of this is due to the increasing use of social links where communication is in shorter and shorter bites, allowing greater and greater chances of misunderstanding with poorer and poorer levels of communication. Further — and this is critical — they generate greater and greater levels of misinformation, at first accidental but later (and to greater and greater degrees) deliberate. The social distancing laws are redefining what it means to 'go to university'. This is all leading to a new pandemic of misinformation.

Revenue shortfalls are driving savage job cuts emphasizing the degree to which universities have been denuded of home-based governmental funds. They emphasize the extent to which overseas student income has become too large a proportion, and the extent to which that amount has been reversed by travel restrictions. Perhaps most recently, they have shown the specific degree to which China is punishing Australia by attempting to dampen Chinese students' desires to come to Australia. In total, it has been estimated that Australia's universities could lose A$5 billion per year over the next few years.

We can compare that figure with the endowments of Australian universities. No Australian university has an endowment larger than A$1.5 billion; most are substantially less. The Australian National University, for example (by some measures the best Australian university) has an endowment of just a little over A$200 million! In contrast, the top ten US universities **each** have endowments totaling **more than US$200 billion**, and even they are hurting!

The overseas student profits were used for what mattered most to the top universities: the 'research rankings arms race'. These institutions are desperate to be seen as international research players, a lot of which is quite stupidly decided. For example, the winning of two Nobel prizes (for one research finding) by one particular university has been sufficient because of the loading applied to a Nobel to push that institution far above its real rank.

Research is expensive. Australian university research has, in recent years, been increasingly underfunded on the basis of OECD comparisons. The entire group of top Australian universities (the group of 8) have just warned that nearly 10,000 of their top researchers in national priority areas are likely to leave for overseas! In lieu of government support, reliance on international students has been the mortgage taken out to fund stellar research reputations, research institutes and buildings.

And though this information applies specifically to research and the group of 8, the effect is far wider.

In 2020, Universities Australia projected that there will be 21,000 job losses across all Australian universities in the next six months. 2021 is proving that to be correct! The government has reduced funding for the higher education sector, and it has specifically excluded public universities from pandemic saver schemes (e.g., JobKeeper). Governments of all colors have been to blame, though the blame seems worst for governments on the right! While the hunger of some universities for dollars is probably almost insatiable, it is certainly convenient to every government that shortfalls were forced by reliance on foreign student earnings.

What Happens Now That the Money Has Stopped?

But we are now past this stage. What happens now that the money has stopped? As it has. The icy fingers of the pandemic chill our best brains as much as they freeze our blocked borders.

Some feel no sympathy for top institutions, which are seen as simply 'down on their luck'. But the problem is a financial pandemic; it is contagious and affecting all universities.

Thus, by taking students they would never previously have accepted, the top universities are trying to make up for the loss of international student funds by swallowing domestic enrolments that would previously have gone to second-level universities. The top-level universities do not really want these students, but they want the money that comes with them! This is draining the enrolment pool of the second-level institutions.

As a result, the second-level institutions are taking students that they too would never have accepted. And this is followed so on, down the line! In the UK, this process already has a name: 'The Hunger Games'.

Further, government needs to create new places for 'new' students. But these new students differ from the new students of prior days. Some are part of the earlier 'baby boom', some are part of the unemployed, work-displaced coronavirus generation, and many are part of the new majority of female students (*who can more easily — it is thought — handle the reduced support and part-time work of today!*).

So, Is There a Solution?

The top universities just want the money. Their real belief is that government should cover their deficits until it is fixed. But who would believe that a blank check to institutions with limitless ambitions and appetites is conceivable?

No politician is that stupid.

That is counter to the mores of government, especially conservative governments.

First, and counterintuitively, the solution must be to save the top institutions intellectually: *'our politicians actually do need to be that stupid'*.

This is necessary because top institutions are the research powerhouses, even if currently they have gone markedly downhill.

Second, it is also essential for *'our politicians to be that stupid'* because just as 'banks were too big to fail', the top universities, in an intellectual sense, should also be 'too good to fail'. To save them intellectually requires saving them financially.

Third, *'our politicians must be that stupid'* because, if the top universities are not saved, they may, by predation, bring down the rest of the educational system with them. This will be catastrophic for whole student generations.

Already for instance, although the top university in Western Australia is in straightened financial straits, its attempt to fix the problem is requiring only a combination of compulsory taking of unpaid leave, pay cuts for many staff and some unhappily accepted redundancies.

In contrast, three other WA universities have announced plans to shed hundreds of staff. One is calling for expressions of interest for voluntary redundancies, with up to 150 redundancies being forced. Another is eyeing a reduction of staff of up to 200. A third is cutting staff numbers by up to 300. These numbers, of course, do not include the work already lost, the casual hours that have already ceased, the terminable contracts that already have been terminated, the positions that have been left unfilled, and the academic areas that have been eliminated.

And these are just the figures for my state. In other words, 'The Hunger Games' has truly started; predation is already occurring.

Fourth, and an order of magnitude greater than all the above, is the effect of the unfortunate bipolar development of the world on Australia. For example, Australia's funding of cybersecurity is supposedly going to be something like **$1.7 billion**. Of this, an almost negligible amount (**$88 million**) is support for education and training in cybersecurity.

Compare this with China, home to the world's most innovative 'cyber-insecurity'. Although China has been 'copying' and 'stealing' intellectual property from abroad for many years, its newer financial inputs into its own educational systems mean that it is now genuinely 'leading' in such education in its own right! We all know that it is still 'stealing', but it now has no need to steal; it is already better than most other systems. Information technology experts have that calculated Australia needs 10 to 100 times as much as committed to be in this race!

21

Are Teaching and Research Careers Now Moribund?

What do you, our young people, think of all this? What do you think about taking careers in research and teaching? Do you think such careers are for you?

Of course, we (the universities) want you. Especially, we want you in all genders, and we particularly want you in STE(A)M (not only science, technology, engineering and medicine, but also including A for art — the creativity of art is part of STEM: an especially important element of research)! But are we still getting you?

Changes for Researchers and Teachers

Research positions for younger people in our universities are increasingly becoming just fixed term positions, and for one to three years only. What used to be excellent research beginnings now lead only to a search for further positions that no longer exist. The next appointees (if the positions are even refilled) start back at the lowest salaries.

Many of these beginning researchers are now becoming aware of the blind alley into which they have strayed.

Let me say immediately that they may have received a good beginning research education. But, more and more, they cannot go further. Among my more recent doctorates, one of the best gave up and moved to industry, which was good for industry but a loss for research. Two others gave up on research careers and went into high school teaching, which was good for the high schools. But it was their second choices. Four more have transitioned to other countries for seriously better research support!

Teaching positions are similarly badly handled. Graduate students, before graduation, can pick up temporary teaching positions, which not only gives them teaching experience but truly helps them to survive during their graduate training. After graduation, there may be a few short-term appointments for teachers of undergraduates, but these disappear at the end of the first postgraduate appointment. The next sequence of teachers starts again at the low first salaries!

The undergraduates, for their part, never seem to realize they are being taught by successive cohorts of beginning teachers who have little experience of teaching.

Let me not knock these beginning teachers. They are often very good. They are close in age to the undergraduates; they have empathy with them; they are up-to-date in the new teaching techniques and information; *and they speak almost the same language*. But they don't yet have disciplinary depth, and the next undergraduate student cohort is taught by a new inexperienced teaching cohort back at square one.

The more experienced teachers who used to form the backbone of teaching scarcely exist at all today. They are costlier, and so have been let go (fired)!

As a result, the principle functions of the university — teaching and research — are being denuded of both already good older people and new good continuing young people.

Why the undergraduates don't complain, I can't understand!

These changes are more fundamental than we realize for four reasons.

Many teachers are now replaced by temporary, part-time teachers.

> *This is the casualization of teachers and teaching!*

Many investigators are now replaced by postdoctoral researchers.

> *This is the 'insecuritization' of researchers and research!*

Many administrators now have academic titles and are 'miscounted' as academics.

> *This is the 'pseudo-academicization' of administrators!*

Many students now have reduced contact with both teachers and researchers.

> *This is the 'invisibilitization' of students!*

Changes for Administrators

In both of the above situations (teaching and research), only those who are lucky(?) enough to pick up beginning administrative positions may be able to move into more continuous career structures. But almost by definition, they are then lost from teaching and research.

Thus, it is mainly university administrators who have positions with a degree of security. It is administration that leads on to more stability and higher salaries, 'escapes' for these 'unwanted academic wannabees'. But of course, this means giving up research and teaching!

Even here there is a trap. Many of the most sought-after administrative positions at the highest levels of all are filled by individuals 'escaping' from universities overseas, particularly from universities in the English-speaking world, especially from the UK itself!

How many deputy vice-chancellors, pro-vice-chancellors and vice-chancellors have themselves been flown in from universities abroad?

Student numbers have increased in the last many years by factors of about 3 to 5 times (entirely reasonable given changes in society). In the same time, administrator numbers have increased by factors of about 5 (or even more).

Teacher and researcher numbers have been reduced, but by how much? Teaching and research appointments are largely insecure. In contrast, university administrators often have 'ongoing appointments', and if they turn out to be not very good for one administrative task, they are not usually 'let go' but are moved to some other task!

Of course, there always were specialist administrators who really knew about financial, staffing and organizational aspects of the university. In England in the old days, these were positions such as bursars, registrars, finance officers, and so on. But the main academic administration in the best universities in the USA was carried out by distinguished professors who were elected (or persuaded) to give a period of administrative service to the university, and who would expect to return afterwards to their disciplines.

In those days, professors were among the academic leaders. They had parking spots! Thus, the highest aim of a young academic was to become a professor and to lead the discipline.

Today, the administration are the leaders. They actually find professors a nuisance. They organize, manage, impose and dispose. They use the methods of the business world. In fairness, of course, much of this has been forced on them, in their turn, by **their** two administrative leaders: *the force of governmental ideologies* and *the reduction of governmental purses*. How career pathways have changed! And as a result, how universities have changed!

Is There an Answer?

How can we improve education?

Perhaps we really ought to apply business principles. When businesses or governments allocate funding to upgrade roads, rails, harbors and airports, they identify, evaluate and prioritize capital investments. Society has rarely invested to upgrade researcher, teacher and servicer supply and quality in the same way as in the bricks-and-mortar projects. Change like this might be a good thing in the current situation.

What is the cost of not doing it? It has been estimated that the difference between a reasonably secure cadre of lifetime-committed academics (researchers, teachers and servicers) and that of temporary, insecure ones could be at least a loss — a capital one — of a million dollars in lifetime earnings per laboratory or classroom. Perhaps to prevent such long-term capital losses, we must start to treat academic activity as a capital investment.

Yet the general antipathy of government toward universities and academia is not driven by long-term vision. In times of scarcity, fear and anxiety in the general notion that universities are places of left-wing views and political correctness, governments think they know how to manage educational policy. They introduce non-evidence-based, short-term policies. And interestingly, though this is worst in politicians of the right, it is evident in the left as well.

The actions they have been taking now will affect our children's future. Let's hope we can influence them to get it right!

22 The World Sphere: Should We be Worried?

In total research and development (R&D) support in various countries (excluding China), the USA tops the list at 45%, with Europe at 25%, near Far East at 17% and South America at 13%. **Australia is at 2%**. Of course, Australia's population is very small. Nevertheless, should Australia worry?

Increases in biomedical R&D spending in recent years have been largely in Asia. China tops the list with an increase of 32.8%. Other Asian countries fall in behind, from South Korea at 11.4%, through Singapore at 10%, India at 6.7% to Japan at 5.7%. In contrast, Europe's spending has increased by 0.4%. USA and Canada's spends are negative at –1.9% and –2.6%. Australia is not in the ballpark at all! Australia's rank order in R&D spending only appears in comparison with some smaller countries (two of which are just city states): Singapore is 7th, Hong Kong 11th, South Korea 14th, and Australia 17th!

Venture capital investment shows the same dismal story. In post- compared with pre-global financial crisis situations, Korea, USA, South Africa and Hungary have all greatly increased their venture capital investments by between 50 to 200%. Australia has reduced it by 60%.

Business collaborations with education in Israel, South Korea, Germany and the United Kingdom have risen by between 25 to 45% in these different countries. Australia's has risen by only 4% in that same time.

Is it not surprising that science, technology and medicine advice to government is dying? No, the advice is not dying, it is the acceptance and use of the advice that is dying!

How about building a sense of trust between citizens and government in the institutions that are there to support them?

How about building a sense of respect for science, technology and medicine, and the facts and expertise inherent within them?

Simple answers will inevitably disappoint. Automatic responses from prepared positions are useless.

Open-minded dialogues, experimental approaches to hard problems and real actions are what are needed. As a society, we must find the imagination and the will!

What is needed has been often expressed by governments. For example, Malcolm Turnbull said that Australia must become a science nation, while Marc Andreesen (in 'It's Time to Build') called for a new spirit of innovation and investment in mathematics, science, technology and medicine. Both called for new products, industries and factories to reboot society.

"Where are the new supersonic aircraft? Where are the millions of delivery drones? Where are the high-speed trains, the soaring monorails, the hyper-loops, and yes, the electric cars, even flying cars? Where are the new medicines, especially the new vaccines, the new anticancer drugs, the new imaging methods, and the new surgeries, together with the new and improved institutions, equipment and personnel, especially the support personnel that go with them? Where are the monies for the large proportion of our society that cannot access these things?"

They have all been described but have never properly eventuated, even though fear of the coronavirus has stimulated incredible activity in 'vaccinology'!

Yet the next plan can't be like the last one! The last one was recognized in Australia years ago by Kevin Rudd. He outlined a broad and growing list of security risks and pressures. Rudd particularly recognized that:

"A pandemic is bound to create real physical, social and policy challenges for Australia."

That statement was made 12 years ago!

Part of Rudd's idea was to include funding and clout for a national security advisor's position in the Prime Minister's department.

This is not unlike the early halcyon days in the UK!

But Tony Abbott quickly abolished that idea. Malcolm Turnbull spoke well about it, but achieved nothing. Scott Morrison has avoided it, removing science inputs from the cabinet!

Many years of reviews, reports and commissions have highlighted the problems facing us. But the rigidities of political ideologies, governmental silos and holding positions conspire to thwart the idea of 'one government', or in other words, to thwart us.

Of course, post-pandemic, Morrison's government is now contemplating a new national security strategy.

This repeats Rudd's ideas of a decade ago.

Will contemplation become action?

First, building national security begins at home. Should we really be relying on others for submarines, face masks, jabs and whatever else?

Second, a strategy without money is rhetorical fluff! The temptation to place too much reliance on 'saving the budget' may continue to intervene (though the pandemic may [temporarily only] scotch that).

Third, there must be coordination, power and funding at the apex of national security: advising in defence, science, technology and medicine.

Fourth, and most critical of all, the intelligence agencies (our contributors to the cyber war) need to be brought into this century, never mind on the way into the next.

Nobel Laureate Joseph Stigler once said:

"We need a better balance between globalization and self-reliance."

But currently the opposite is evident. The modern globalization cycle has faced a series of blows from increasing US isolation on almost every front, the European debt crisis, the UK Brexit farce and the US-China trade and nationalism wars, as well as the increasing rise of populisms, separatisms and tribalisms in many countries.

Australia has had only small parts to play here, though it does have specifically Australian elements: droughts, fires and floods. But all of these are still waiting, a year and more later, for real help. Do we have to wait for a 'war-time atmosphere' in which fundamental change suddenly seems possible? Or are we just waiting to return to business as usual?

Have we arrived at a position where ideology can be put on one side, and a genuine collaboration across the public and private sectors can emerge? Is this what modern government should be all about — totally focused on challenge, using all elements of collaboration, no more dreaded silos?

Should all this worry us?

Yet greater than all the above threats are separate developments in China. China has enormously increased all aspects of its university industry. The numbers of higher education institutions in China has risen from 2,300 to 2,700 in just the last five years. The number of Chinese universities in the top 100 in the world has risen from 1 to 20 in that time. The quality of research in China has changed from the earlier copying and stealing of external ideas and machinery (which nevertheless still goes on) to creating its own new knowledge and better machines. There was a time was when the most powerful computers were in the USA, some twenty times more powerful than those in China. Now, the best computers are Chinese (see another chapter). Even the business of stealing information is done so much better, with enormously more funding, by China than by any other country in the world. Although China has the strongest knowledge-espionage system, it actually no longer needs to rely on it. In China, what is home-grown is becoming the best.

As a result, China is changing from educating its best young people by sending them abroad to doing it at home. One estimate of the fall in overseas Chinese education is an estimated reduction by 2030 of almost 75% of the 2020 level in the overseas education of Chinese students.

The world has had universities for more than two millennia. No business, government or nation has survived for so long. This is because universities have been different, separate from businesses, governments and nationalities. Universities have allowed independent voices, independent thoughts, independent actions and independent machines to flourish.

In my youth in the UK, changes in education in the 1950s gradually resulted in a far greater number of individuals being able to access higher education. The peak of this followed from the Robbins Report that created many new universities in the UK and led over the following years to higher education being available from, previously, some 4 percent of the student population to as much as 40 percent. In so doing, however it started the process of embedding rigidity into the educational process, of deinvesting in higher learning, and of replacing collegiality with managerialism. More universities, yes, but reduced funding per institution.

In my mid-life in the USA, changes in higher education have, of course, been far more frequent, as well as far more complex, due to the complicated nature of US higher education itself, especially its wide variety as a result of the combination of federal, state local, private and religious institutions. Since the 1970s in the USA, a concatenation of changes has resulted in enormously increased costs of education for students and student families, and in enormously reduced resources, especially of staff, for the institutions themselves. Despite rising tuition rates, top professorial positions have gradually been replaced with poorly paid part-time positions and graduate-student casual labor. Community colleges and for-profit colleges rely almost exclusively on adjunct teachers. Today, these (and other factors) are resulting in the closure of large numbers of lower level institutions.

In Australia in the 1990s, following the Dawkins report, there was reduced funding per institution. Costello, then Abbot, and finally Morrison, all caused more university damage. Most recently, Morrison's damage is especially visible because of the misfortune of Covid-19 magnifying the standard liberal anti-university (therefore anti-liberal — in its old-fashioned meaning) stance!

These various damages in the UK, USA and Australia did not occur in parallel. As indicated, they started earliest in the UK, somewhat later in the USA, and only in the last three decades or so in Australia.

Today in the UK, these changes have resulted in some 30,000 jobs at risk and a reduction of £2.6 billion in funding. In the USA, 650,000 jobs (13 percent of the workforce) have gone. Australia has lost 17,000 research positions, together with continued reductions not only of full time staff, but interestingly also of part-time staff. Increases have been recorded only for casual staff! Despite the powers of Google, it is difficult to obtain full information about these numbers!

In general, our western societies and governments tend to blame these damages on the failure of internal university governance processes. They seem not to realize that these internal processes are constrained, even forced, by external government funding reductions. University executives can scarcely be anything other than undemocratic.

Yet these enforced staff reductions and high staff casualizations pose major risks to the quality of higher education delivery and the adequate support of student growth, experiences and outcomes. The effects of special reductions of senior academic leaders and of broad fields of endeavor especially reduce quality in teaching and learning, research and practice, and, especially, their interactions.

Paradoxically, the most recent damages from the effects of the pandemic coronavirus may be pointing to a way out. Thus, educational, scientific, technological, medical and even more general advices normally asked for and provided to (but largely ignored and even rejected by) governments are starting to be accepted again in the face of public and governmental fear engendered by the pandemic. Governments everywhere are so alarmed, even frightened, that they are actually asking for, listening to, and sometimes following the advices that they are receiving. We likely will manage our way out of this disaster by applying these advices. But will we have really learnt the lesson? Or will we then return to isolationisms, populisms, tribalisms, nationalisms and separatisms?

It is now time to return to the purpose of this
book as outlined on the first page:

for the young, dreaming about where they are going,

for parents, especially physician and scientist parents, wondering if
their children should follow them,

for grandparents of all kinds, thinking about
chances for grandchildren,

for everyone, interested in teaching, discovery, service
and challenging,

and for everyone, seeking change and desiring improvement.

Let us examine these points in reverse. My generations (retired grandparents, even great-grandparents) enjoyed our academic and professional work enormously. We participated in the many research developments of those years. We had no hesitation in supporting our children in following similar careers.

The current generations (mid-career parents, many of whom are physicians, scientists and teachers) initially also enjoyed their careers and gave us the fantastic research developments of the present. But they have also become aware of the recent deleterious changes.

"I was trained to be a doctor, not an accountant,"

they say, as they take up early retirement! They now wonder if their offspring should follow.

The new generations (today's schoolies, undergraduates, post-graduates, aspiring teachers, new researchers and young practitioners) are now dreaming about where they should go. These new generations are especially in position to understand how research, teaching and practice really occur. This is why, although I want you, I have also presented you with the problems.

It is now up to you, the next many years of would-be-educated people, to save the system by doing what we did not, challenging successfully both inside and outside. It is rather like the climate concatenation: the young will have to save us from ourselves. Again, I can think of no better advice than to modify the words of Edson Arantes do Nascimento (Pelé):

Acredita No Veio. Listen to *this* Old Man.

9 789811 264191